DAVIS'S
DRUG
GUIDE
for NURSES®
EIGHTEENTH EDITION

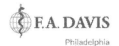

F.A. DAVIS

Philadelphia

ISBN: 978-7-7469-0065-8

NURSING PHARMACOLOGY

Nursing, calling that takes care of the nonstop consideration of the wiped out, the harmed, the debilitated, and the withering. Nursing is additionally answerable for empowering the soundness of people, families, and networks in clinical and local area settings. Medical attendants are effectively engaged with medical services research, the board, strategy thoughts, and patient backing. Medical attendants with postbaccalaureate arrangement take care of giving essential medical care and specialty administrations to people, families, and networks.

Proficient medical attendants work both freely and as a team with other medical care experts like doctors. Proficient medical attendants administer crafted by attendants who have restricted licenses, like authorized down to earth medical attendants (LPNs) in the US and enlisted medical caretakers (ENs) in Australia. Proficient attendants additionally supervise crafted by nursing aides in different settings.

Nursing is the biggest, the most assorted, and one of the most regarded of all the medical services callings. There are more than 2.9 million enrolled medical caretakers in the US alone, and a lot more millions around the world. While genuine segment portrayal stays a tricky objective, nursing has a higher relative portrayal of racial and ethnic minorities than other medical services callings. In certain nations, nonetheless, men actually remain fundamentally underrepresented.

The interest for nursing stays high, and projections propose that such interest will considerably increment. Propels in medical services innovation, rising assumptions for individuals looking for care, and redesign of medical care frameworks require a more prominent number of profoundly taught experts. Segment changes, like huge maturing populaces in numerous nations of the world, additionally fuel this interest.

History of nursing

Albeit the beginnings of nursing originate before the mid-nineteenth hundred years, the historical backdrop of expert nursing generally starts with Florence Songbird. Songbird, the knowledgeable girl of well off English guardians, resisted social shows and chose to turn into a medical caretaker. The nursing of outsiders, either in emergency clinics or in their homes, was not then seen as a decent vocation for very much reproduced women, who, on the off chance that they wished to nurture, were supposed to do so just for wiped out family and close companions. In an extreme takeoff from these perspectives, Songbird trusted that knowledgeable ladies, utilizing logical standards and informed training about sound ways of life, could emphatically work on the consideration of wiped out patients. Besides, she accepted that nursing gave an ideal autonomous calling brimming with scholarly and social opportunity for ladies, who around then had not many other vocation choices.

In 1854 Songbird had the potential chance to test her convictions during England's Crimean War. News stories revealing that debilitated and injured Russian warriors breast fed by strict orders fared far superior to English troopers aroused popular assessment. Accordingly, the English government requested that Songbird take a little gathering of medical caretakers to the tactical clinic at Scutari (cutting edge Üsküdar, Turk.). Not long after their appearance, Songbird and her attendants had redesigned the encampment clinic as per nineteenth century science: walls were cleaned for sterilization, windows opened for ventilation, supporting food arranged and served, and meds and medicines productively regulated. Inside the space of weeks demise rates dove, and troopers were not generally nauseated by irresistible illnesses emerging from poor clean circumstances. Inside the space of months a thankful public knew about crafted by the "Woman with the Light," who made daily adjusts encouraging the debilitated and injured. Toward the finish of the nineteenth 100 years, the whole Western world shared Songbird's faith in the value of taught medical attendants.

Songbird's accomplishments eclipsed alternate ways of nursing the wiped out. For a really long time, most nursing of the debilitated had occurred at home and had been the obligation of families, companions, and regarded local area individuals with notorieties as powerful healers. During plagues, like cholera, typhus, and smallpox, men took on dynamic nursing jobs. For instance, Stephen Girard, a well off French-conceived financier, won the hearts of residents of his took on city of Philadelphia for his gutsy and sympathetic nursing of the survivors of the 1793 yellow fever pandemic.

As urbanization and industrialization spread, those without families to really focus on them ended up in medical clinics where the nature of nursing care shifted gigantically. A few patients got incredible consideration. Ladies from strict nursing orders were especially known for the nature of the nursing care they gave in the clinics they laid out. Different medical clinics relied upon recuperating patients or employed people for the nursing care of patients. Once in a while this care was fantastic; different times it was lamentable, and the untrustworthiness of clinic based nursing care turned into a specific issue by the late nineteenth 100 years, when changes in clinical practices and medicines required equipped medical attendants. The combination of emergency clinics' necessities, doctors' desires, and ladies' craving for significant work prompted another medical services proficient: the prepared attendant.

Medical clinics laid out their own preparation schools for attendants. In return for addresses and clinical directions, understudies furnished the clinic with a few years of talented free nursing care. This clinic based instructive model had huge long haul suggestions. It bound the instruction of medical caretakers to emergency clinics instead of universities, a tie that was not conclusively broken until the last 50% of the twentieth 100 years. The clinic based preparing model likewise supported isolation in the public eye and in the medical care framework. For example, African American understudy attendants were banned from practically all American clinics and preparing schools. They could look for preparing just in schools laid out by African American medical clinics. In particular, the medical clinic based preparing model reinforced the social generalizing of nursing as ladies' work. A couple of medical clinics gave preparing to keep up with men's conventional jobs inside nursing.

In any case, medical caretakers changed clinics. Notwithstanding the gifted, merciful consideration they provided for patients, they laid out a methodical, daily schedule, and systemized climate inside which patients mended. They managed progressively muddled medicines and prescription systems. They kept up with the aseptic and disease control conventions that permitted more complicated and obtrusive medical procedures to continue. Moreover, they explored different avenues regarding various models of nursing mediations that acculturated progressively specialized and unoriginal operations.

Outside emergency clinics, prepared nurture immediately became basic in the battle against irresistible illnesses. In the mid twentieth 100 years, the newfound "microorganism hypothesis" of sickness (the information that numerous ailments were brought about by microbes) caused extensive alert in nations all over the planet. Showing strategies for forestalling the spread of illnesses, like tuberculosis, pneumonia, and flu, turned into the area of the meeting attendants in the US and the region medical caretakers in the Unified Realm and Europe. These medical attendants really focused on contaminated patients in the patients' homes and helped families and networks the actions important to forestall spreading the disease. They were especially dedicated to working with poor and migrant networks, which frequently had little admittance to other medical care administrations. Crafted by these medical caretakers added to a sensational decrease in the mortality and dismalness rates from irresistible illnesses for youngsters and grown-ups.

Simultaneously, self-employed entities called private-obligation medical attendants really focused on debilitated people in their homes. These attendants performed significant clinical work and upheld families who had the monetary assets to manage the cost of care, yet the unregulated medical services work market left them defenseless against rivalry from both undeveloped medical attendants and every year's class of recently graduated prepared attendants. Very soon, the stock of private-obligation medical caretakers was more prominent than the interest from families. At the turn of the twentieth hundred years, medical caretakers in industrialized nations started to lay out proficient relationship to set principles that separated crafted by prepared attendants from both assistive-nursing staff and undeveloped attendants. More significant, they effectively looked for permitting security for the act of enlisted nursing. Later on, attendants in certain nations went to aggregate bartering and work associations to help them in affirming their and their patients' freedoms to further develop conditions and make quality nursing care conceivable.

By the mid-1930s the rising mechanical and clinical requests of patient consideration, the raising requirements of patients for escalated nursing, and the subsequent development of such consideration out of homes and into emergency clinics requested clinic staffs of prepared as opposed to understudy attendants. By the mid-1950s clinics were the biggest single boss of enlisted attendants. These pattern proceeds, in spite of the fact that as changes in medical services frameworks have reemphasized care at home, a proportionately more noteworthy number of attendants work in short term centers, home consideration, general wellbeing, and other local area based medical services associations.

Other significant changes in nursing happened during the last 50% of the twentieth 100 years. The calling developed more different. For instance, in the US, the Public Association of Hued Graduate Medical caretakers (NOCGN) profited by the intense lack of attendants during The Second Great War and effectively pushed for the integration of both the tactical nursing corps and the nursing affiliations. The American Medical attendants Affiliation (ANA) integrated in 1949, perhaps the earliest public expert relationship to do as such.

Thus, in 1951, feeling its objectives satisfied, the NOCGN broke up. However, by the last part of the 1960s a few African American medical caretakers felt that the ANA had neither the time nor the assets to address every one of their interests sufficiently. The Public Dark Medical caretakers Affiliation (NBNA) shaped in 1971 as an equal association to the ANA.

Nursing's instructive design additionally different. Reliance on emergency clinic based preparing schools declined, and those schools were supplanted with university programs either in local area or specialized universities or in colleges. Likewise, more methodical and inescapable projects of graduate instruction started to arise. These projects plan attendants for jobs in administration and schooling as well as for jobs as clinical trained professionals and medical caretaker specialists. Nurture no longer needed to look for doctoral certificates in fields other than nursing. By the 1970s attendants were laying out their own doctoral projects, underscoring the nursing information and science and exploration expected to address squeezing nursing endlessly care conveyance issues.

During the final part of the twentieth hundred years, medical attendants answered rising quantities of wiped out patients with inventive rearrangements of their examples of care. For instance, basic consideration units in clinics started when medical caretakers began gathering their most fundamentally sick patients to give more successful utilization of present day innovation. What's more, explores different avenues regarding models of moderate patient consideration and essential nursing reemphasized the obligation of one medical attendant for one understanding notwithstanding the frequently overpowering administrative requests by clinics on medical caretakers' time.

The nursing calling likewise has been reinforced by its rising accentuation on public and worldwide work in agricultural nations and by its promotion of solid and safe conditions. The global extent of nursing is upheld by the World Wellbeing Association (WHO), which perceives nursing as the foundation of most medical services frameworks all over the planet.

The act of nursing

Extent of nursing practice

As per the Worldwide Committee of Attendants (ICN), the extent of nursing practice "envelops independent and cooperative consideration of people of any age, families, gatherings, and networks, wiped out or well and in all settings." Public nursing affiliations further explain the extent of nursing practice by laying out specific practice norms and sets of principles. Public and state organizations likewise control the extent of nursing practice. Together, these bodies put forward legitimate boundaries and rules for the act of medical attendants as clinicians, instructors, chairmen, or analysts.

Instruction for nursing practice

Attendants enter practice as generalists. They care for people and groups of any age in homes, clinics, schools, long haul care offices, short term centers, and clinical workplaces. Numerous nations expect three to four years of instruction at the college level for generalist practice, in spite of the fact that varieties exist. For instance, in the US, medical caretakers can enter generalist practice through a two-year program in a junior college or a four-year program in a school or college.

Groundwork for specialization in nursing or high level nursing practice generally happens at the expert's level. A school or college degree in nursing is expected for access to most dominate's projects. These projects accentuate the evaluation and the board of ailments, pharmacology, wellbeing schooling, and administered practice in specialty fields, like pediatrics, psychological well-being, ladies' wellbeing, local area wellbeing, or geriatrics.

Research readiness in nursing happens at the doctoral level. Coursework underlines nursing information and science and exploration techniques. A unique and meaningful exploration study is expected for finish of the doctoral certification.

Types of general nursing practice

Medical clinic based nursing practice

Medical clinic nursing is maybe the most natural of all types of nursing practice. Inside emergency clinics, in any case, there are a wide range of kinds of practices. A few medical caretakers care for patients with sicknesses like diabetes or cardiovascular breakdown, while others care for patients previously, during, and after medical procedure or in pediatric, mental, or labor units. Medical attendants work in mechanically modern basic consideration units, like escalated care or cardiovascular consideration units. They work in crisis divisions, working rooms, and recuperation rooms, as well as in short term centers. The talented consideration and solace medical caretakers give patients and families are just a piece of their work. They are additionally liable for training people and families ways of overseeing ailments or wounds during recuperation at home. At the point when essential, they train patients ways of adapting to ongoing circumstances. Most clinic based medical caretakers are generalists. Those with cutting edge nursing degrees give clinical oversight and meeting, work in administration, and lead patient-care research.

Local area wellbeing nursing practice

Local area wellbeing nursing consolidates differing titles to depict crafted by medical attendants in local area settings. Over the course of the last hundreds of years and in various areas of the planet, local area wellbeing attendants were called region medical attendants, visiting medical attendants, general wellbeing medical attendants, home-care medical caretakers, and local area wellbeing attendants. Today people group wellbeing nursing and general wellbeing nursing are the most widely recognized titles utilized by attendants whose practices center around advancing and safeguarding the strength of populaces. Information from nursing, social, and general wellbeing sciences illuminates local area wellbeing nursing rehearses. In numerous nations, guaranteeing that required wellbeing administrations are given to the most helpless and hindered bunches is vital to local area wellbeing nursing practice. In the US, people group wellbeing attendants work in different settings, including state and nearby wellbeing offices, school wellbeing programs, transient wellbeing facilities, neighborhood wellbeing focuses, senior focuses, word related wellbeing programs, nursing focuses, and home consideration programs. Care at home is many times considered to be a favored option for really focusing on the debilitated. Today home-care attendants give extremely refined, complex consideration in patients' homes. Universally, home consideration is being inspected as an answer for the requirements of the developing quantities of older requiring care.

Psychological well-being nursing practice

Psychological well-being (or mental) nursing practice focuses on the consideration of those with profound or stress-related concerns. Medical caretakers practice in ongoing units of emergency clinics or in short term emotional wellness centers, and they work with people, gatherings, and families. High level practice psychological well-being attendants additionally give psychotherapy to people, gatherings, and families in confidential practice, talk with local area associations to give psychological well-being backing, and work with different medical caretakers in both long term and short term settings to meet the feelings of patients and families battling with actual diseases or wounds.

The consideration of kids

The consideration of kids, frequently alluded to as pediatric nursing, centers around the consideration of babies, youngsters, and teenagers. The consideration of families, the main help in children's' lives, is likewise a fundamentally significant part of the consideration of kids.

Pediatric medical caretakers work to guarantee that the typical formative requirements of youngsters and families are met even as they work to treat the side effects of difficult ailments or wounds. These medical attendants likewise work to advance the soundness of kids through vaccination programs, youngster misuse mediations, dietary and actual work instruction, and wellbeing screening drives. Both generalist and expert pediatric medical attendants work in clinics, short term facilities, schools, day-care focuses, and elsewhere kids are to be found.

The consideration of ladies

The consideration of ladies, particularly of childbearing and childrearing ladies (frequently called maternal-kid nursing), has for quite some time been a specific nursing concern. As soon as the 1920s, attendants worked with public and neighborhood states, confidential foundations, and other concerned experts to guarantee that moms and kids got appropriate nourishment, social help, and clinical consideration. Afterward, attendants started working with public and global organizations to ensure privileges to sufficient medical care, regard for basic liberties, insurance against savagery, admittance to quality regenerative wellbeing administrations, and dietary and instructive help. Generalist and expert medical attendants really focusing on ladies work on obstetrical and gynecological units in clinics and in an assortment of short term centers, clinical workplaces, and strategy sheets. Many have specific mastery in such regions as osteoporosis, bosom taking care of help, aggressive behavior at home, and emotional wellness issues of ladies.

Geriatric nursing practice

Geriatric nursing is one of the quickest developing areas of nursing practice. This development matches segment need. For instance, projections in the US propose that more drawn out futures and the effect of the "time of increased birth rates" age will bring about a huge expansion in the quantity of people over age 65. In 2005 people north of 65 represented around 13% of the complete populace; be that as it may, they are supposed to represent very nearly 20% of the absolute populace by 2030. In addition, those north of 65 utilize more medical care and nursing administrations than some other segment bunch. Most schools of nursing consolidate explicit substance on geriatric nursing in their educational programs. Progressively, all generalist medical attendants are ready to really focus on old patients in different settings including medical clinics, short term centers, clinical workplaces, nursing homes, restoration offices, helped residing offices, and people's own homes. Experts focus on additional particular parts of senior consideration, including keeping up with capability and personal satisfaction, conveying psychological wellness administrations, offering natural help, overseeing drugs, lessening the dangers for issues, for example, falling, disarray, skin breakdown, and contaminations, and taking care of the moral issues related with slightness and weakness.

High level nursing practice

Nurture experts

Nurture experts are ready at the expert's level in colleges to give a wide scope of symptomatic and treatment administrations to people and families. This type of cutting edge nursing practice started in the US during the 1960s, following the section of medical services regulation (Federal medical insurance and Medicaid) that reliable residents over age 65 and low-pay residents admittance to medical services administrations. Accordingly, a few medical caretakers, working in a joint effort with doctors, got extra preparation and extended their training by taking care of the conclusion and therapy of normal intense and stable persistent sicknesses of youngsters and grown-ups. At first, nurture specialists worked in essential consideration settings; there they treated basically solid youngsters who experienced routine colds, contaminations, or formative issues, performed actual tests on grown-ups, and worked with the two people and families to guarantee side effect steadiness in such sicknesses as diabetes, coronary illness, and emphysema. Today nurture professionals are a significant part of essential medical care administrations, and their training has ventured into specialty regions also. Particular attendant experts frequently work in a joint effort with doctors in trauma centers, concentrated care units of emergency clinics, nursing homes, and clinical practices.

Clinical nursing subject matter experts

Clinical nursing experts are ready in colleges at the expert's level. Their clinically engaged schooling is specifically strengths, like nervous system science, cardiology, restoration, or psychiatry. Clinical nursing experts might furnish direct consideration to patients with complex nursing needs, or they might give conference to generalist medical caretakers. Clinical nursing experts likewise direct proceeding with staff schooling programs. They normally work in emergency clinics and short term facilities, albeit some clinical nursing experts lay out free practices.

Nurture maternity specialists

Nurture maternity specialists are established in the exceptionally old practice of labor at home. Maternity specialists, as opposed to obstetricians, have generally been the essential supplier of care to birthing ladies, and they remain so in many pieces of the industrialized and creating world. In the US during the 1930s, a few attendants started consolidating their abilities with those of maternity specialists to offer birthing ladies options in contrast to obstetrical consideration. The new specialty of medical attendant birthing assistance developed gradually, serving for the most part poor and geologically burdened ladies and their families. The ladies' development starting during the 1960s got a flood interest for nurture birthing specialists from ladies who needed both the effortlessness of a customary conveyance and the wellbeing of accessible innovation in the event that any issues created. Quantities of medical attendant birthing assistants in the US developed from less than 300 out of 1963 to north of 7,000 out of 2007. Today most medical caretaker birthing assistants are ready in colleges at the expert's level. They convey almost 300,000 children consistently, and, rather than customary maternity specialists, who convey in homes, nurture maternity specialists do so basically in clinics and formal birthing communities. Worldwide interest for nurture birthing assistance care is projected to essentially develop.

Nurture anesthetists

Nurture anesthetists started rehearsing in the late nineteenth 100 years. Prepared medical caretakers, who around then were turning into an undeniably significant presence in working rooms, took care of both controlling sedation and giving individualized patient checking to any responses during surgeries. Nurture anesthetists demonstrated their worth during The Second Great

War, when they were the sole suppliers of sedation in every tactical emergency clinic. Today nurture anesthetists are laid out medical services suppliers. In the US alone they give 66% of all sedation benefits and are the sole suppliers of sedation administrations in most provincial American medical clinics. Nurture anesthetists train at the postgraduate level, either in expert's projects in schools of nursing or in associated programs in branches of wellbeing sciences. They work wherever sedation is conveyed: in working rooms, obstetrical conveyance suites, wandering careful focuses, and clinical workplaces.

Authorizing

Given the basic significance of normalized and safe nursing care, all nations have laid out systems for guaranteeing negligible capabilities for section into training and keeping on nursing instruction. Those nations with unified wellbeing frameworks, like numerous European and South American nations, sanction public frameworks for nurture authorizing. Nations with decentralized and privatized frameworks, for example, the US surrender to states and areas the power to decide negligible attendant authorizing necessities. In many cases licenses are time-restricted and can be repudiated assuming conditions warrant such an activity. Authorizing recharging frequently relies upon some strategy for confirming proceeded with ability.

Public associations

In basically every nation of the world, there is a public nursing association that advances principles of training, advocates for safe patient consideration, and verbalizes the calling's situation on squeezing medical services issues to strategy sheets, government organizations, and the overall population. Numerous public nursing associations additionally have related diaries that broadcast research discoveries, disperse convenient clinical data, and talk about results of strategy drives. What's more, most nursing strength and high level practice bunches have their own associations and related diaries that contact both public and worldwide crowds. There are a wide assortment of nursing specific vested parties. Various associations additionally participate in aggregate haggling and work coordinating for medical attendants.

Global associations

The Worldwide Gathering of Medical caretakers (ICN), an organization of north of 128 public attendants affiliations situated in Geneva, represents nursing universally. The World Wellbeing Association (WHO) has had a well-established interest in advancing the job of nursing, especially as free local area based suppliers of essential medical care in Third World and other underserved nations. The Global Board of the Red Cross (ICRC) and its public associates has long perceived the basic job of nursing in misfortune help and continuous wellbeing training projects.

The investigation of pharmacology centers around the utilization of medications and their job in forestalling and treating illnesses. The consequences for the body, like secondary effects, drug co-operations, and unfavorable responses, are parts of pharmacology studies. Nursing requires an exhaustive comprehension of pharmacology as it is necessary to the training.

Job of Nursing Pharmacology

Attendants incorporate the investigation of pharmacology into their training to give prescription administration and forestall unfriendly occasions. A comprehension of pharmacology permits attendants to really play out the accompanying assignments.

Pharmacology

Pharmacology, part of medication that arrangements with the communication of medications with the frameworks and cycles of living creatures, specifically, the systems of medication activity as well as the helpful and different purposes of the medication.

The primary Western pharmacological composition, a posting of home grown plants utilized in old style medication, was made in the first century Promotion by the Greek doctor Dioscorides. The clinical discipline of pharmacology gets from the archaic pharmacists, who both arranged and recommended drugs. In the mid nineteenth century a split created between pharmacists who treated patients and those whose interest was essentially in the readiness of restorative builds; the last option shaped the premise of the creating specialty of pharmacology. A genuinely logical pharmacology grew solely after propels in science and science in the late eighteenth century empowered medications to be normalized and sanitized. By the mid nineteenth 100 years, French and German scientific experts had confined numerous dynamic substances — morphine, strychnine, atropine, quinine, and numerous others — from their rough plant sources. Pharmacology was solidly settled in the later nineteenth hundred years by the German Oswald Schmeiderberg (1838-1921). He characterized its motivation, composed a reading material of pharmacology, served to establish the main pharmacological diary, and, in particular, headed a school at Strasbourg that turned into the core from which free divisions of pharmacology were laid out in colleges all through the world. In the twentieth hundred years, and especially in the years since The Second Great War, pharmacological exploration has fostered a huge swath of new medications, including anti-toxins, like penicillin, and numerous hormonal medications, like insulin and cortisone. Pharmacology is by and by engaged with the improvement of additional compelling renditions of these and a huge range of different medications through compound union in the research center. Pharmacology additionally looks for additional proficient and compelling approaches to managing drugs through clinical exploration on enormous quantities of patients.

How Do Stomach settling agents Work?

During the mid-twentieth hundred years, pharmacologists became mindful that a connection exists between the substance design of a compound and the impacts it produces in the body. Since that time, expanding accentuation has been put on this part of pharmacology, and concentrates regularly portray the progressions in drug activity coming about because of little changes in the substance construction of the medication. Since most clinical mixtures are natural synthetics, pharmacologists who participate in such examinations should fundamentally have a comprehension of natural science.

Significant fundamental pharmacological examination is done in the exploration labs of drug and synthetic organizations. After 1930 this area of pharmacological exploration went through a huge and fast development, especially in the US and Europe.

Crafted by pharmacologists in industry manages the thorough tests that should be made prior to promising new medications can be brought into clinical use. Nitty gritty perceptions of a medication's impacts on all frameworks and organs of research center creatures are essential before the doctor can precisely foresee both the impacts of the medication on patients and their likely poisonousness to people overall. The pharmacologist doesn't himself test the impacts of medications in patients; this is done solely after comprehensive tests on creatures and is generally directed by doctors to decide the clinical viability of new medications. Steady testing is additionally expected for the normal control and normalization of medication items and their intensity and immaculateness.

Receptor 2 Bad guy: Conventional and Brand Names

Here is a table of the most usually utilized H2 bad guys.

Receptor 2 adversaries (closes in - tidine)

cimetidine (Tagamet)

ranitidine (Zantac)

famotidine (Pepcid)

nizatidine (Axid)

Depiction

Receptor 2 bad guys block the arrival of hydrochloric corrosive in light of gastrin.

These medications incorporate cimetidine (Tagamet), ranitidine (Zantac), famotidine (Pepcid), and nizatidine (Axid).

Remedial activities

The ideal activities of H2 bad guys incorporate the accompanying:

Specifically block H2 receptors situated on the parietal cells.

Forestalls the arrival of gastrin, a chemical that causes nearby arrival of receptor (because of feeling of receptor receptors), eventually hindering the creation of hydrochloric corrosive.

Diminishes pepsin creation by the central cells.

Sign

Receptor 2 adversaries are shown for the accompanying:

Transient treatment of dynamic duodenal ulcer or harmless gastric ulcer.

Treatment of obsessive hyper-secretory conditions like Zollinger-Ellison disorder (obstructing the overproduction of hydrochloric corrosive that is related with these circumstances).

Prophylaxis of stress-actuated ulcers and intense upper GI draining in basic patients (impeding the creation of corrosive safeguards the stomach lining, which is in danger as a result of diminished bodily fluid creation related with intense pressure).

Treatment of erosive gastroesophageal reflux (diminishing the corrosive being spewed into the throat will advance recuperating and decline torment).

Help of side effects of indigestion, corrosive heartburn, and sharp stomach.

Contraindications and Alerts

The contraindications and alerts while utilizing H2 adversaries include:

Sensitivity. The H2 adversaries ought not be utilized with known aversion to any medications of this class to forestall extreme touchiness responses.

Pregnancy or lactation. Wariness ought to be utilized during pregnancy or lactation due to the potential for unfavorable consequences for the embryo or nursing child.

Hepatic or renal brokenness. Mindfulness ought to be utilized in patients with hepatic or renal brokenness, which could impede drug digestion and discharge.

Drawn out or nonstop use. Care ought to likewise be taken assuming drawn out or nonstop utilization of these medications is important in light of the fact that they might be veiling serious basic circumstances.

Antagonistic impacts

The unfriendly impacts related with H2 adversaries are:

CNS: Dazedness, disarray, cerebral pain, drowsiness.

Cardio: Heart arrhythmias, heart failure.

GI: Loose bowels.

Regenerative: Barrenness.

Skin: Rash.

Misc: Gynecomastia.

Collaborations

Cimetidine, famotidine, and ranitidine can dial back the digestion of the accompanying medications, prompting expanded serum levels and conceivable poisonous responses:

- Warfarin.
- Enemies of coagulants.
- Phenytoin.
- Beta-adrenergic blockers.
- Liquor.
- Quinidine.
- Lidocaine.
- Theophylline.
- Chloroquine.
- Benzodiazepines.
- Nifedipine.
- Pentoxifylline.
- TCAs.
- Procainamide.
- Carbamazepine.

Nursing Contemplations

Nursing contemplations for a patient utilizing H2 bad guys incorporate the accompanying:

Nursing Appraisal

Nursing evaluation for a patient utilizing H2 bad guys include:

Survey for potential contraindications and alerts: history of sensitivity to any H2 bad guys to forestall expected unfavorably susceptible responses; hindered renal or hepatic capability, which could influence the digestion and discharge of the medication; a definite portrayal of the GI issue, including time span of the problem and clinical assessment to assess the fitting utilization of the medication and probability of hidden clinical issues; and current status of pregnancy and lactation in view of the potential for unfriendly consequences for the hatchling or infant.

Carry out an actual assessment to lay out gauge information prior to starting treatment, decide viability of the treatment, and assess for any unfriendly impacts related with drug treatment.

Examine the skin for proof of sores or rash to screen for antagonistic responses.

Assess neurological status, including direction and influence, to evaluate CNS impacts of the medication and to make arrangements for defensive measures.

Survey cardiopulmonary status, including beat, circulatory strain, and electrocardiogram (in the event that IV use is required), to assess the cardiovascular impacts of the medication.

Carry out stomach assessment, including evaluation of the liver, to lay out a standard and preclude basic clinical issue.

Screen the aftereffects of research center tests, including liver and renal capability tests, to anticipate changes in digestion or discharge of the medication that could require portion change.

Nursing Determination

Nursing determination connected with the medication treatment could incorporate the accompanying:

Intense agony connected with CNS and GI impacts.

Upset tangible discernment (sensation, hear-able) connected with CNS impacts.

Diminished cardiovascular result connected with heart arrhythmias.

Risk for injury connected with CNS impacts.

Lacking information in regards to tranquilize treatment.

Nursing Care Plans and Mediations

Nursing intercessions for patients utilizing H2 bad guys include:

Guarantee remedial levels. Manage drug with or before feasts and at sleep time (precise timing differs with item) to guarantee remedial levels when the medication is generally required.

Forestall serious poisonousness. Set up for diminished portion in instances of hepatic or renal brokenness to forestall serious poisonousness.

Screen IV dosages cautiously. Screen the patient constantly if giving IV portions to permit early location of possibly serious unfavorable impacts, including cardiovascular arrhythmias

Evaluate for potential medication drug collaborations. Survey the patient cautiously for any potential medication drug co-operations whenever given in blend with different medications due to the medications impacts on liver compound frameworks.

Give patient's solace. Give solace, including analgesics, prepared to get to washroom offices, and help with ambulation, to limit conceivable antagonistic impacts.

Reorient patient completely. Intermittently reorient the patient and organization wellbeing measures on the off chance that CNS impacts happen to guarantee patient security and endlessly work on understanding resistance of the endlessly drug impacts.

Go to standard subsequent meet-ups. Set up for customary development to assess drug impacts and the basic issues.

Offer help. Offer help and support to assist patients with adapting to the illness and the medication routine.

Instruct the client. Give patient educating with respect to tranquilize name, dose, and timetable for organization; significance of dispersing organization fittingly as requested; need for promptly accessible admittance to washroom; signs and side effects of unfriendly impacts and measures to limit or forestall them.

Assessment

Assessment of a patient utilizing H2 bad guys include:

Screen patient reaction to the medication (help of GI side effects, ulcer recuperating, and counteraction of movement of ulcer).

Screen for unfavorable impacts (tipsiness, disarray, mental trips, GI adjustments, cardiovascular arrhythmias, hypotension, and gynecomastia).

Assess the viability of the showing plan (patient can name drug, dose, unfriendly impacts to look for, and explicit measures to stay away from them).

Screen the adequacy of solace measures and consistence with the routine.

As an attendant, it is critical to have an exhaustive comprehension of different drugs to give the best consideration to patients. This article intends to give an itemized outline of albuterol signs and helpful impacts. From its purposes in treating asthma and constant obstructive pneumonic sickness (COPD) to its viability in forestalling exercise-prompted bronchospasm, albuterol assumes an imperative part in overseeing respiratory problems. We should dive into the numerous features of albuterol and investigate its helpful advantages.

What is Albuterol?

Albuterol, likewise realized by its image names Ventolin or Proventil, is a generally endorsed prescription used to treat different respiratory circumstances. It is a short-acting beta-agonist bronchodilator drug that works by loosening up the smooth muscles in the aviation routes. It acts explicitly on the beta-2 receptors in the lungs, prompting the enlargement of the bronchioles and improvement in wind stream. Albuterol is accessible in different structures, including inhalers, nebulizers, tablets, and syrups.

Nonexclusive Name

Albuterol, otherwise called salbutamol, is the nonexclusive name of the prescription. The nonexclusive name addresses the dynamic fixing in the medication, which is liable for its helpful impacts.

Brand Names

Albuterol is showcased under different brand names, contingent upon the drug organization producing and conveying the prescription. A portion of the notable brand names for albuterol incorporate Ventolin, Proventil, ProAir, and AccuNeb. These brand names might change in various nations and locales.

Drug Order of Albuterol

Albuterol is named a short-acting beta-agonist (SABA). It has a place with the class of medications known as beta-2 adrenergic agonists or bronchodilators.

Restorative Class

bronchodilators

Pharmacologic Class

adrenergics

Signs and Restorative Impacts

Albuterol is fundamentally demonstrated for the treatment and the executives of asthma and COPD. This part will zero in on examining the assorted remedial impacts of albuterol in reducing respiratory side effects and further developing lung capability.

1. Asthma. Albuterol is regularly recommended for people with asthma. It is successful in easing intense bronchospasm, an unexpected tightening of the aviation routes that makes breathing troublesome. Albuterol goes about as a bronchodilator, loosening up the muscles around the aviation routes and permitting more straightforward wind stream. It gives prompt alleviation during asthma assaults and helps control constant side effects.

2. Work out Initiated Bronchospasm (EIB). A few people experience bronchospasm during actual work. Albuterol can be utilized as a preventive measure before exercise to diminish the probability

of bronchospasm and further develop practice resistance. By opening up the aviation routes, it empowers people with EIB to participate in proactive tasks with decreased respiratory side effects.

3. COPD. Albuterol is additionally helpful for people with COPD, including constant bronchitis and emphysema. It gives alleviation from bronchospasms and further develops lung capability. Albuterol's bronchodilatory impacts assist with broadening the aviation routes, making it simpler to inhale and lessening side effects like hacking and windedness.

4. Bronchiolitis. Albuterol might be utilized as a feature of the treatment plan for babies and little youngsters with bronchiolitis, a viral contamination that influences the little aviation routes in the lungs. It can assist with reducing aviation route aggravation and work on respiratory side effects in these cases.

5. Cystic Fibrosis. Albuterol can help with slackening and cleaning bodily fluid off of the aviation routes in people with cystic fibrosis, in this manner further developing lung capability and decreasing the gamble of respiratory diseases.

6. Indicative Device. Albuterol is in many cases used in bronchodilator challenge tests to assess aviation route hyper-responsiveness and affirm the determination of asthma or COPD. These tests include estimating lung capability when the organization of albuterol to survey the patient's reaction.

System of Activity

Albuterol applies its belongings by restricting to the beta-2 adrenergic receptors found on the smooth muscles coating the aviation routes in the lungs. This limiting actuates the receptors, prompting the excitement of a catalyst called adenylate cyclase. Adenylate cyclase changes over adenosine triphosphate (ATP) into cyclic adenosine monophosphate (cAMP), which initiates protein kinase A (PKA). Enactment of PKA brings about the unwinding of the smooth muscles encompassing the aviation routes, prompting bronchodilation and further developed wind stream.

The instrument of activity of albuterol includes the accompanying advances:

1. Receptor Actuation. Albuterol specifically ties to the beta-2 adrenergic receptors, which are available principally in the aviation route smooth muscle cells.

2. Feeling of Adenylate Cyclase. Restricting of albuterol to the beta-2 receptors initiates a compound called adenylate cyclase. This actuation prompts the transformation of adenosine triphosphate (ATP) into cyclic adenosine monophosphate (cAMP).

3. Expanded cAMP Levels. Raised degrees of cAMP inside the smooth muscle cells enact protein kinase A (PKA), a chemical that controls different cell processes.

4. Muscle Unwinding. PKA phosphorylates proteins engaged with muscle constriction, prompting unwinding of the smooth muscles encompassing the aviation routes. This unwinding brings about bronchodilation, which extends the aviation routes and considers further developed wind stream.

Safety measures and Contraindications

While albuterol is for the most part protected and successful when utilized as coordinated, there are sure safety measures and contraindications to consider. It is critical to know about these prior to beginning albuterol treatment.

Safety measures

1. Sensitivities. People ought to illuminate their medical services supplier on the off chance that they have a known sensitivity to albuterol or some other prescriptions. Hypersensitive responses to albuterol are uncommon yet can happen, prompting side effects like rash, tingling, expanding, or trouble relaxing.

2. Cardiovascular Circumstances. People with a background marked by heart issues, for example, heart beat problems, coronary conduit illness, or hypertension, ought to examine their condition with their medical services supplier. Albuterol can increment pulse and circulatory strain, and its utilization in people with extreme cardiovascular circumstances might require cautious assessment of dangers and advantages.

3. Diabetes. People with diabetes ought to intently screen their glucose levels while utilizing albuterol, as it might influence glucose digestion.

Changes in diabetes the board might be important under the direction of a medical services supplier.

4. Thyroid Issues. People with thyroid circumstances, like hyperthyroidism or hypothyroidism, ought to illuminate their medical care supplier. Albuterol might possibly influence thyroid capability and may require cautious checking in such cases.

5. Seizure Issues. People with a background marked by seizures ought to examine their condition with their medical services supplier prior to utilizing albuterol. Albuterol can at times cause quakes or intensify existing seizure problems.

6. Pregnancy and Breastfeeding. Pregnant people, those wanting to become pregnant, or breastfeeding people ought to counsel their medical services supplier prior to utilizing albuterol. The possible dangers and advantages of albuterol during pregnancy or lactation ought to be painstakingly assessed.

Contraindications

1. Excessive touchiness. Albuterol is contraindicated in people who have a known excessive touchiness or sensitivity to albuterol or

any of its parts. Unfavorably susceptible responses to albuterol can go from gentle skin responses to serious fundamental responses, including hypersensitivity.

2. Extreme Cardiovascular Circumstances. Albuterol can invigorate the heart and increment pulse and circulatory strain. Consequently, it is contraindicated in people with serious cardiovascular circumstances, like unsound or extreme coronary illness, including myocardial dead tissue (respiratory failure) inside the new period, and extreme arrhythmias.

3. Pregnancy-prompted Hypertension. Albuterol ought to be utilized with alert or stayed away from in people with pregnancy-prompted hypertension (toxemia or eclampsia). The medicine's expected impacts on circulatory strain can additionally muddle these circumstances.

4. Shut point Glaucoma. Albuterol is contraindicated in people with shut point glaucoma, a kind of glaucoma where the liquid in the eye can't deplete as expected. Albuterol can cause pupillary enlargement, which can worsen the condition and lead to an unexpected expansion in intraocular pressure.

5. Hyperthyroidism. Albuterol might possibly demolish side effects in people with hyperthyroidism, a condition portrayed by an overactive thyroid organ. It is contraindicated in people with uncontrolled hyperthyroidism.

6. Attendant Use with Monoamine Oxidase Inhibitors (MAOIs). Albuterol ought not be utilized simultaneously with or in something like fourteen days of ceasing treatment with MAOIs. The blend of albuterol and MAOIs can prompt a hypertensive emergency, a serious expansion in pulse.

Drug Co-operations

Albuterol, similar to any prescription, can cooperate with different medications, normal items, and certain food sources. These communications might modify the viability of albuterol or increment the gamble of aftereffects. It is essential to know about potential medication collaborations with albuterol.

Drug-Medication

1. Beta-Blockers. Simultaneous utilization of albuterol with non-particular beta-blockers, for example, propranolol, can repress the

bronchodilator impacts of albuterol. Beta-blockers can alienate the activity of albuterol on beta-2 adrenergic receptors, prompting diminished bronchodilation and possibly deteriorating respiratory side effects.

2. Diuretics. Certain diuretics, like circle diuretics (e.g., furosemide), can drain potassium levels in the body. Albuterol, being a beta-2 adrenergic receptor agonist, can likewise diminish potassium levels. Simultaneous utilization of albuterol with diuretics might expand the gamble of hypokalemia (low potassium levels). Standard observing of potassium levels is significant in such cases.

3. Other Sympathomimetic Specialists. Joining albuterol with other sympathomimetic specialists, like different bronchodilators or decongestants, might possibly prompt an added substance impact, expanding the gamble of cardiovascular aftereffects like expanded pulse and circulatory strain.

Drug-Regular Items

1. Home grown Enhancements. A few home grown supplements, for example, ephedra or mama huang, have energizer properties that can increment pulse and circulatory strain.

Simultaneous utilization of these enhancements with albuterol might upgrade the cardiovascular impacts of albuterol, expanding the gamble of unfavorable impacts.

2. Caffeine. High caffeine admission, for example, from espresso, tea, or caffeinated drinks, might possibly expand the energizer impacts of albuterol, prompting expanded pulse and apprehension. Restricting caffeine utilization while utilizing albuterol to limit potential aftereffects is prudent.

Drug-Food

1. Grapefruit Juice. Grapefruit juice can restrain the protein liable for the digestion of specific drugs, including albuterol. This can build the degrees of albuterol in the body, possibly prompting an expanded gamble of aftereffects. Abstaining from drinking grapefruit juice while taking albuterol is prudent.

2. High-Fat Dinners. Utilization of high-fat dinners can defer the retention of albuterol, bringing about a postponed beginning of activity. It is for the most part prescribed to take albuterol while starving or as guided by the medical care supplier to guarantee ideal ingestion and adequacy.

Unfriendly Impacts

Normal Secondary effects:

1. Quakes. One of the most normally detailed symptoms of albuterol is gentle quakes or shaking of the hands. These quakes are by and large transitory and die down after some time as the body acclimates to the prescription.

2. Expanded Pulse. Albuterol can cause an expansion in pulse, known as tachycardia. This impact is generally gentle and transient, yet people with previous heart conditions might be more vulnerable to encountering a fast pulse.

3. Palpitations. A few people might encounter a vibe of sporadic or strong pulses, known as palpitations while utilizing albuterol. In the event that palpitations are serious or tenacious, counseling a medical care provider is significant.

4. Anxiety and Fretfulness. Albuterol can incidentally cause sensations of apprehension, fretfulness, or nervousness. These impacts are by and large gentle and transitory.

5. Migraine. Migraines are a potential symptom of albuterol. In the event that migraines become

extreme or persevering, looking for clinical attention is fitting.

More uncommon Aftereffects:

1. Muscle Issues. A few people might encounter muscle cramps while utilizing albuterol. Guaranteeing appropriate hydration and electrolyte equilibrium might assist with mitigating these side effects.

2. Tipsiness. Albuterol can cause tipsiness or wooziness in certain people. It is critical to utilize alert while performing exercises that require sharpness.

3. A sleeping disorder. Trouble dozing or a sleeping disorder might happen as a result of albuterol. Taking albuterol prior in the day and trying not to even portions might assist with limiting rest aggravations.

Unfriendly Responses:

1. Hypersensitive Responses. Indications of a hypersensitive response to albuterol incorporate rash, tingling, enlarging (particularly of the face, lips, tongue, or throat), extreme dazedness, or

trouble relaxing. Hypersensitivity, a serious unfavorably susceptible response, is a health related crisis and requires prompt clinical consideration.

2. Chest Torment. Chest torment or distress might happen as an interesting unfavorable response to albuterol. It is critical to look for sure fire clinical consideration assuming that chest torment happens while utilizing albuterol.3. Demolishing Breathing Issues. At times, albuterol may strangely cause deteriorating breathing troubles, for example, expanded wheezing, windedness, or hacking.

Organization Contemplations

Accessible Structures

Tablets: 2 mg, 4 mg.

Expanded discharge tablets: 4 mg, 8 mg.

Oral syrup (strawberry-seasoned): 2 mg/5 mL.

Metered-portion spray: 90 mcg/inward breath in 6.7-g, 8-g, 8.5-g, and 18-g canisters (200 metered inward breaths), 100 mcg/shower.

Inward breath arrangement: 0.63 mg/3 mL (0.021%), 1.25 mg/3 mL (0.042%), 2.5 mg/3 mL (0.083%), 1 mg/mL, 2 mg/mL, 5 mg/mL (0.5%).

Powder for inward breath (Proair Respiclick): 90 mcg/inward breath (200 metered inward breaths).

Powder for inward breath (Ventolin Diskus): 200 mcg.

In blend with: ipratropium (Combivent, DuoNeb).

Measurements for Youngsters

Inhaln (Youngsters): 1.25 mg/portion q 8 hr by means of nebulization or 1 - 2 puffs through MDI into the ventilator circuit q 6 hrs.

Measurements for Youngsters

PO (Youngsters ≥12 yr): 2 - 4 mg 3 - multiple times day to day (not to surpass 32 mg/day) or 4 - 8 mg of expanded discharge tablets two times every day.

PO (Kids 6-12 yr): 2 mg 3-4 times day to day or 0.3 - 0.6 mg/kg/day as broadened discharge tablets partitioned two times every day; might be painstakingly expanded on a case by case basis (not to surpass 8 mg/day).

PO (Kids 2 - 6 yr): 0.1 mg/kg multiple times day to day (not to surpass 2 mg multiple times every day at first); might be painstakingly expanded to 0.2

mg/kg multiple times day to day (not to surpass 4 mg multiple times day to day).

Inhaln (Kids ≥4 yr): Through metered-portion inhaler — 2 inward breaths q 4 - 6 hr or 2 inward breaths 15 min before work out (90 mcg/shower); a few patients might answer 1 inward breath. NIH Rules for intense asthma worsening: Youngsters — 4 - 8 puffs q 20 min for 3 dosages then q 1-4 hr; Grown-ups — 4-8 puffs q 20 min for up to 4 hr then q 1-4 hr prn.

Inhaln (Youngsters >12 yr): Through dry powder inhaler — 2 inward breaths q 4 - 6 hr or 2 inward breaths 15 - 30 min before work out (90 mcg/shower); a few patients might answer 1 inward breath q 4 hr.

Inhaln (Youngsters >12 yr): NIH Rules for intense asthma compounding by means of nebulization or IPPB — 2.5-5 mg q 20 min for 3 dosages then 2.5 - 10 mg q 1 - 4 hr prn; Persistent nebulization — 10 - 15 mg/hr.

Inhaln (Youngsters 2 - 12 yr): NIH Rules for intense asthma compounding by means of nebulization or IPPB — 0.15 mg/kg/portion (least portion 2.5 mg) q 20 min for 3 dosages then 0.15 - 0.3 mg/kg (not to exceed 10 mg) q 1-4 hr prn or

1.25 mg 3-4 times every day for kids 10-15 kg or 2.5 mg 3-4 times day to day for youngsters

---

15 kg; Nonstop nebulization — 0.5 - 3 mg/kg/hr.

Measurement for Grown-ups

PO (Grown-ups): 2 - 4 mg 3 - multiple times every day (not to surpass 32 mg/day) or 4 - 8 mg of expanded discharge tablets two times day to day.

Inhaln (Grown-ups): Through metered-portion inhaler — 2 inward breaths q 4 - 6 hr or 2 inward breaths 15 min before work out (90 mcg/splash); a few patients might answer 1 inward breath. NIH Rules for intense asthma compounding: Youngsters — 4 - 8 puffs q 20 min for 3 dosages then q 1-4 hr; Grown-ups — 4-8 puffs q 20 min for up to 4 hr then q 1-4 hr prn.

Inhaln (Grown-ups): By means of dry powder inhaler — 2 inward breaths q 4 - 6 hr or 2 inward breaths 15 - 30 min before work out (90 mcg/shower); a few patients might answer 1 inward breath q 4 hr.

Inhaln (Grown-ups): NIH Rules for intense asthma compounding by means of nebulization or IPPB — 2.5-5 mg q 20 min for 3 portions then 2.5 - 10 mg q 1 - 4 hr prn; Ceaseless nebulization — 10 - 15 mg/hr.

Measurements for Geriatric Patients

PO (Geriatric Patients): Introductory portion shouldn't surpass 2 mg 3 - multiple times every-day, might be expanded cautiously (up to 32 mg/day).

Pharmacokinetics

1. Retention. Albuterol is accessible in different structures, including inhalers (metered-portion inhalers or dry powder inhalers) and oral tablets/syrup. When breathed in, albuterol is quickly retained through the respiratory mucosa and arrives at the lungs straightforwardly, giving a fast beginning of activity. The oral definition is assimilated from the gastrointestinal lot and goes through some level of first-pass digestion in the liver.

2. Dispersion. Albuterol has a moderate volume of dissemination, demonstrating that it is dispersed all through the body tissues. It promptly crosses cell layers, including the blood-mind hindrance, and is circulated into the focal sensory system. Albuterol

is insignificantly bound to plasma proteins, permitting it to be accessible for activity.

3. Digestion. Albuterol goes through digestion essentially in the liver. The significant pathway includes sulfate and glucuronide formation, prompting the arrangement of dormant metabolites. The metabolites are essentially wiped out by means of the kidneys.

4. Disposal. Albuterol and its metabolites are principally killed through the kidneys by means of renal discharge. The disposal half-existence of albuterol is roughly 3 to 6 hours, meaning it requires this measure of investment for half of the medication fixation to diminish in the body.

Extraordinary Populaces:

1. Pediatric Patients. The pharmacokinetics of albuterol might change in pediatric patients, particularly babies. Cautious portion change and observing might be fundamental in this populace.

2. Old Patients. Old patients might encounter more slow leeway of albuterol because old enough related changes in renal capability. Portion changes in view of individual reaction might be required.

3. Renal or Hepatic Disability. People with renal or hepatic disability might have modified pharmacokinetics of albuterol. Close checking and portion change are fundamental in these cases.

Nursing Contemplations for Albuterol

While really focusing on patients getting albuterol, medical attendants assume a critical part in observing their reaction to the drug and guaranteeing protected and compelling therapy. Here are significant nursing contemplations:

Nursing Appraisal

Nursing appraisals are not just vital in the underlying phases of drug organization yet in addition all through the patient's treatment process. By leading careful appraisals, attendants can accumulate important data about the patient's wellbeing status, reaction to drug, and generally progress. This empowers them to pursue informed choices, give fitting consideration, and team up successfully with different individuals from the medical care group.

1. Evaluate respiratory status of patient.

Observing the patient's respiratory rate assesses the adequacy of albuterol in working on relaxing.

Changes in respiratory rate might show the requirement for additional mediation or change in the prescription routine.

2. Auscultate patient's breath sounds.

Auscultating breath sounds permits medical attendants to evaluate the viability of albuterol in alleviating bronchospasm. Unusual breath sounds, for example, wheezing or lessened breath sounds, may demonstrate the requirement for extra mediations or changes in the treatment plan.

3. Screen patient's oxygen immersion.

Checking oxygen immersion levels through beat oximetry surveys the patient's oxygenation status and the reaction to albuterol treatment. Enhancements in oxygen immersion show the viability of the drug in upgrading oxygen trade.

4. Survey patient's pulse.

Albuterol can make cardiovascular impacts, including expanded pulse. Routinely evaluating the patient's pulse distinguishes any progressions that might be connected with the medicine and takes into consideration convenient intercession if necessary.

5. Survey patient's pulse.

Checking the patient's circulatory strain is essential to assess cardiovascular security during albuterol treatment. Tremendous changes in circulatory strain, like hypertension or hypotension, may require further appraisal and joint effort with the medical services supplier.

6. Evaluate patient for sensitivities.

Evaluating the patient's sensitivities is pivotal to recognize any potential touchiness responses to Albuterol or related prescriptions. This data guarantees patient security and guide fitting medicine decisions.

7. Survey patient's drug history.

Gathering data about the patient's medicine history distinguishes potential medication collaborations or contraindications that might impact the organization of albuterol. This evaluation guarantees the protected and successful utilization of the drug.

8. Evaluate patient's clinical history.

Grasping the patient's clinical history, including any prior respiratory or cardiovascular circumstances, supports fitting the organization and observing of albuterol to meet their particular requirements. It recognizes expected gambles and illuminates the treatment plan.

9. Survey patient's mental status.

Albuterol treatment can at times cause anxiety or tension as a secondary effect. Surveying the patient's mental status recognizes any progressions in mind-set or uneasiness levels, considering suitable help and mediation if necessary.

10. Evaluate patient's adherence to drug routine.

Reasoning: Surveying the patient's adherence to the endorsed Albuterol routine is significant for assessing treatment viability. This appraisal recognizes any obstructions or difficulties the patient might look in sticking to the drug plan and considers proper training and backing.

Albuterol Nursing Intercessions

Here are some nursing intercessions for patients getting albuterol:

1. Direct albuterol as recommended.

Albuterol is a bronchodilator used to treat respiratory circumstances. Controlling the prescription as recommended guarantees that the patient gets the restorative impacts of the medicine and further develops aviation route leeway.

2. Instruct the patient on legitimate inhaler method.

Right inhaler procedure is essential for ideal medicine conveyance. Showing the patient the legitimate strategy guarantees that they get the full portion of albuterol, boosting its adequacy in alleviating bronchospasm.

3. Note changes in respiratory status routinely.

Standard checking of respiratory status surveys the patient's reaction to albuterol treatment. It considers early identification of changes in respiratory rate, breath sounds, and oxygen immersion, empowering brief mediation if necessary.

4. Screen for medicine aftereffects.

Albuterol can cause incidental effects like quakes, apprehension, and fast pulse. Checking for these secondary effects distinguishes any unfavorable responses and takes into account proper administration or change of the prescription routine if vital.

5. Screen for drug co-operations.

Albuterol might cooperate with different drugs, like beta-blockers or monoamine oxidase inhibitors (MAOIs). Evaluating the patient's drug history and talking with the medical services supplier distinguishes possible co-operations and forestall difficulties.

6. Screen pulse and circulatory strain.

Albuterol can make cardiovascular impacts, including expanded pulse and changes in circulatory strain. Consistently checking these fundamental signs distinguishes any irregularities and takes into account ideal intercession or meeting with the medical care supplier.

7. Instruct the patient on likely unfavorably susceptible responses.

A people might have sensitivities or excessive touchiness to albuterol. Teaching the patient about expected unfavorably susceptible responses and training them to report any signs or side effects of a hypersensitive reaction guarantees early acknowledgment and fitting administration.

8. Give schooling on the significance of drug adherence.

Albuterol is much of the time utilized on a planned premise to oversee respiratory circumstances. Teaching the patient about the significance of sticking to the recommended measurement and timetable enhances treatment results and forestall intensifications.

9. Work together with the medical services group for individualized care.

Working together with the medical services group, including doctors, respiratory advisors, and drug specialists, guarantees far reaching and individualized care for patients getting albuterol. It considers facilitated endeavors in streamlining treatment and tending to a particular patient requirements or concerns.

10. Screen the patient's reaction to albuterol treatment.

Consistently assessing the patient's reaction to Albuterol treatment decides the viability of the prescription and guides further mediations or changes in the treatment plan depending on the situation.

Patient Training and Instructing

Here are some understanding instruction and lessons for patients getting albuterol:

1. Show appropriate inhaler strategy.

Showing the patient how to utilize the inhaler accurately guarantees that they get the full portion of albuterol and expands its adequacy in easing bronchospasm. Legitimate method incorporates appropriate hand situating, inward breath coordination, and breath holding.

2. Make sense of the reason and activity of albuterol.

Giving an unmistakable clarification of why albuterol is recommended and the way that it works assists the patient with understanding its job in dealing with their respiratory condition. This understanding advances prescription adherence and enables the patient to partake in their consideration effectively.

3. Stress the significance of medicine adherence.

Albuterol is much of the time utilized on a planned premise to oversee respiratory circumstances. Focusing on the significance of accepting the drug as endorsed guarantees ideal treatment results, forestalls intensifications, and further develops in general infectious prevention.

4. Talk about expected secondary effects and the board procedures.

Illuminating the patient about conceivable symptoms of albuterol, like quakes, anxiety, and fast pulse, helps them expect and deal with these impacts. Giving methodologies, for example, unwinding strategies or revealing serious aftereffects advances patient solace and security.

5. Show the patient how to perceive and answer intensifications.

Instructing the patient on the signs and side effects of deteriorating respiratory pain or intensifications assists them with distinguishing when to immediately look for clinical help. Brief intercession can forestall entanglements and diminish the requirement for crisis care.

6. Talk about the significance of trying not to triggers and oversee ecological variables.

Numerous respiratory circumstances, like asthma, can be set off or demolished by specific ecological elements. Instructing the patient about normal triggers and methodologies for evasion, for example, allergen control or smoking end, advances illness the board and decreases intensifications.

7. Give composed directions to medicine organization and dose plan.

Composed directions act as a source of perspective for the patient, guaranteeing exact self-organization and measurements adherence. This lessens the gamble of mistakes and builds up the data gave during verbal instructing.

8. Address different kinds of feedback the patient might have.

Empowering an open exchange permits the patient to communicate any vulnerabilities or nerves they might have in regards to albuterol or their respiratory condition. Resolving their different kinds of feedback advances figuring out, consistence, and by and large persistent fulfillment.

9. Include relatives or guardians in the educating system.

Reasoning: Including relatives or guardians establishes a steady climate for the patient. Teaching them about the patient's respiratory condition, albuterol organization, and perceiving potential entanglements upgrades the general consideration and wellbeing of the patient.

10. Plan follow-up visits for progressing checking and assessment.

Customary subsequent visits permit medical care suppliers to evaluate the patient's reaction to albuterol treatment, address any worries or changes in side effects, and make essential acclimations to the therapy plan. This guarantees progressing ideal consideration and illness the board.

Assessment and Wanted Results

1. Further developed Aviation route Leeway. Albuterol plans to assuage bronchospasm and

work with better wind current, bringing about superior aviation route leeway and diminished respiratory trouble.

2. Diminished Respiratory Side effects. The ideal result is a decrease in respiratory side effects like hacking, wheezing, windedness, and chest snugness. Albuterol ought to assist with lightening these side effects, permitting the patient to inhale all the more serenely.

3. Improved Breathing Example. Albuterol ought to work on the patient's breathing example by diminishing respiratory rate, further developing lung capability, and advancing viable inward breath and exhalation.

4. Expanded Oxygenation. The ideal result is further developed oxygenation, as proven by an expansion in oxygen immersion levels. Albuterol improves oxygen trade in the lungs, prompting better oxygenation of the blood and tissues.

5. Further developed Exercise Resilience. Albuterol expects to improve the patient's activity resistance by decreasing activity instigated bronchospasm. The ideal result is the capacity to participate in proactive tasks with negligible respiratory limits or side effects.

6. Decreased Dependence on Salvage Drug. Albuterol ought to assist with limiting the requirement for salvage drugs, like short-acting bronchodilators, by giving supported alleviation from respiratory side effects and decreasing the recurrence of intensifications.

7. Counteraction of Respiratory Confusions. The ideal result is a diminishing in the event and seriousness of respiratory confusions, for example, asthma assaults or intensifications of ongoing obstructive pneumonic sickness (COPD). Albuterol plans to actually forestall and deal with these inconveniences.

8. Worked on Personal satisfaction. Albuterol treatment ought to prompt a superior personal satisfaction for patients by lessening respiratory side effects, improving actual work, and permitting them to participate in day to day exercises without huge constraints or uneasiness.

9. Limited Hospitalizations and Trauma center Visits. The ideal result is a diminishing in the requirement for medical clinic confirmations and trauma center visits connected with respiratory intensifications. Albuterol expects to give viable side effect control, forestalling extreme respiratory

episodes and decreasing the requirement for intense clinical consideration.

10. Patient Fulfillment. Eventually, the ideal result shows restraint fulfillment with the adequacy of albuterol in dealing with their respiratory condition. Patient criticism and announced improvement in side effects are significant marks of fruitful treatment.

What is Furosemide?

Furosemide, ordinarily realized by its image name Lasix, is a diuretic prescription broadly utilized in the treatment of different circumstances like edema (liquid maintenance) and hypertension (hypertension). It has a place with a class of medications called circle diuretics and works by expanding how much pee created by the kidneys, consequently assisting with taking out overabundance liquid and diminish enlarging. It is accessible in oral tablet structure, as well as in injectable plans for intravenous use in hospitalized patients. Furosemide works by hindering the reabsorption of sodium, chloride, and water in the kidneys, prompting expanded pee creation. This diuretic impact assists with decreasing liquid over-burden in the body, alleviating side effects like expanding, windedness, and hypertension.

Nonexclusive Name

Furosemide is the nonexclusive name for this diuretic drug. The dynamic fixing gives restorative impacts and is available in both the brand-name and conventional forms of the medication.

Brand Names

Lasix is one of the ordinarily perceived brand names for furosemide. It is a deeply grounded and generally involved brand that has been available for a long time. While there are other brand names for furosemide, Lasix has earned notoriety and respect among medical care experts and patients the same.

Drug Arrangement of Furosemide

The medication grouping of furosemide is:

Helpful Class

Furosemide has a place with the helpful class of diuretic prescriptions. Diuretics are drugs that advance diuresis, which is the expanded creation of pee. They are ordinarily recommended to treat conditions described by liquid maintenance, like edema (expanding) and hypertension (hypertension). By expanding pee yield, diuretics help to eliminate abundance liquid from the body, lessening enlarging and bringing down pulse.

Pharmacologic Class

Inside the class of diuretics, furosemide explicitly falls under the subclass of circle diuretics. This class of diuretics gets its name from the site of activity inside the kidneys where they apply their belongings, explicitly the circle of Henle. Circle diuretics like furosemide work by hindering the reabsorption of sodium, chloride, and water in this piece of the renal tubules, prompting expanded pee creation and resulting disposal of overabundance liquid from the body.

Signs and Restorative Impacts

Furosemide tracks down application in different ailments, including:

1. Edema related with cardiovascular breakdown. Cardiovascular breakdown is an ongoing condition portrayed by the heart's powerlessness to productively siphon blood. This can bring about liquid amassing in various pieces of the body, prompting edema. Furosemide is frequently endorsed to lessen liquid over-burden and free side effects like expanding and brevity from breath.

2. Hypertension. Furosemide is in some cases utilized as adjunctive treatment in the treatment of hypertension. By advancing diuresis, it assists with diminishing blood volume and thusly lower circulatory strain. In any case, it is essential to take note of that furosemide alone isn't viewed as a first-line treatment for hypertension and is regularly utilized in mix with other antihypertensive specialists.

3. Renal disability. In patients with kidney issues, for example, intense renal disappointment or constant kidney sickness, furosemide might be recommended to upgrade diuresis and forestall liquid over-burden. By expanding pee yield, it can assist with eliminating side-effects and poisons from the body, further developing kidney capability.

4. Liver cirrhosis. Liver cirrhosis is a condition portrayed by irreversible scarring of the liver tissue, which can prompt liquid gathering in the midsection (ascites). Furosemide is frequently utilized as a feature of the administration procedure for ascites to advance diuresis and diminish stomach expanding.

5. Pneumonic edema. Pneumonic edema alludes to the collection of liquid in the lungs, frequently brought about by conditions like congestive cardiovascular breakdown or intense respiratory trouble disorder. Furosemide might be managed to assist with taking out overabundance liquid from the lungs and work on relaxing.

Instrument of Activity

Furosemide applies its restorative impacts by focusing on a particular vehicle protein called the Na-K-2Cl cotransporter, which is liable for the reabsorption of sodium, chloride, and potassium particles in the thick rising appendage of the circle of Henle in the kidneys. By restraining this carrier, furosemide forestalls the reabsorption of these particles, prompting expanded discharge in the pee.

This component of activity advances diuresis as well as influences the equilibrium of electrolytes in the body. Furosemide can cause expanded discharge of potassium, magnesium, and calcium particles, which might require supplementation to keep up with ordinary levels and forestall electrolyte lopsided characteristics.

Safety measures and Contraindications

While considering the utilization of furosemide, it is essential to know about the precautionary measures and contraindications related with this diuretic prescription. These rules assist with guaranteeing the protected and suitable utilization of furosemide in people with different ailments. Here are the precautionary measures and contraindications to consider:

Furosemide Precautionary measures

While furosemide is a compelling diuretic prescription, it is essential to know about specific precautionary measures while utilizing this medication. Insurances are rules and contemplations that should be considered to guarantee the protected and suitable utilization of the drug. Here are a few significant precautionary measures to remember:

1. Sensitivities. People with known aversions to furosemide or other sulfonamide drugs ought to practice alert. Hypersensitive responses might incorporate skin rashes, tingling, enlarging, or trouble relaxing. It is critical to educate medical services suppliers regarding any sensitivities prior to starting therapy.

2. Kidney Capability. Furosemide fundamentally influences kidney capability. People with debilitated kidney capability or a background marked by kidney illness ought to utilize furosemide with alert. Measurements changes might be important to guarantee protected and compelling use.

3. Electrolyte Irregular characteristics. Furosemide can cause changes in electrolyte levels, including potassium, sodium, and magnesium. Standard observing of electrolyte levels is significant, particularly for people with prior electrolyte awkward nature or conditions like cardiovascular breakdown or liver infection.

4. Diabetes. Furosemide can influence glucose levels and may require changes in the administration of diabetes. Close observing of blood glucose levels is significant for people with diabetes who are taking furosemide.

5. Pregnancy and Breastfeeding. Pregnant or breastfeeding people ought to counsel their medical services suppliers prior to utilizing furosemide. The likely dangers and advantages of the prescription should be painstakingly assessed in these circumstances.

6. Other Ailments. People with specific ailments, like liver sickness, gout, lupus, or electrolyte irregularities, ought to illuminate their medical care suppliers prior to beginning furosemide therapy. Close observing and conceivable portion changes might be fundamental.

Furosemide Contraindications

Contraindications are explicit circumstances or conditions in which the utilization of prescription isn't suggested or ought to be stayed away from altogether. For furosemide, coming up next are significant contraindications to know about:

1. Sensitivity to Sulfonamide Drugs. Furosemide has a place with the sulfonamide class of medications. People with a known sensitivity to sulfonamide prescriptions ought to try not to utilize furosemide, as it might prompt a hypersensitive response.

2. Anuria. Anuria, the powerlessness to deliver pee, is a contraindication for furosemide use. Since furosemide depends on pee creation to apply its diuretic impacts, it won't be viable in people with anuria.

3. Serious Electrolyte Lopsided characteristics. Furosemide is contraindicated in people with serious electrolyte lopsided characteristics, for example, seriously low potassium or sodium levels. The utilization of furosemide might demolish this awkward nature.

4. Hypovolemia. People with serious hypovolemia, a huge lessening in blood volume, shouldn't utilize furosemide. Furosemide advances diuresis, which further lessens blood volume and can compound the condition.

5. Hepatic Trance like state. Furosemide is contraindicated in people with hepatic trance like

state, an extreme liver condition portrayed by loss of cognizance and liver disappointment.

Drug Collaborations

While utilizing furosemide, it is critical to know about potential medication communications that can happen. Drug co-operations can influence the manner in which meds work in the body, prompting decreased adequacy or expanded chance of aftereffects. Here are some normal medication co-operations related with furosemide:

Drug-Medication

1. Nonsteroidal Mitigating Medications (NSAIDs). NSAIDs, like ibuprofen and naproxen, can lessen the diuretic and antihypertensive impacts of furosemide. Simultaneous use ought to be observed, and measurement changes might be important.

2. Lithium. Furosemide can expand the disposal of lithium from the body, possibly decreasing its viability in overseeing temperament issues. Close observing of lithium levels and changes in measurement might be required.

3. Different Diuretics. Simultaneous utilization of furosemide with different diuretics can potentiate

the diuretic impact and increment the gamble of lack of hydration and electrolyte awkward nature. Alert is encouraged, and close observing of electrolyte levels is vital.

4. Corticosteroids. Furosemide can upgrade the potassium-exhausting impacts of corticosteroids, prompting an expanded gamble of hypokalemia. Normal checking of potassium levels and change of treatment might be fundamental.

5. Digoxin. Furosemide can modify the degrees of digoxin in the body, possibly expanding the gamble of digoxin harmfulness. Close observing of digoxin levels and proper dose changes are significant.

Drug Communications

While utilizing furosemide, it is critical to know about potential medication connections that can happen. Drug connections can influence the manner in which prescriptions work in the body, prompting decreased adequacy or expanded chance of aftereffects. Here are some normal medication collaborations related with furosemide:

Drug-Medication

1. Nonsteroidal Mitigating Medications (NSAIDs). NSAIDs, like ibuprofen and naproxen, can lessen the diuretic and antihypertensive impacts of furosemide. Simultaneous use ought to be observed, and measurement changes might be vital.

2. Lithium. Furosemide can expand the end of lithium from the body, possibly lessening its adequacy in overseeing mind-set issues. Close observing of lithium levels and changes in measurements might be required.

3. Different Diuretics. Simultaneous utilization of furosemide with different diuretics can potentiate the diuretic impact and increment the gamble of lack of hydration and electrolyte awkward nature. Alert is encouraged, and close observing of electrolyte levels is vital.

4. Corticosteroids. Furosemide can upgrade the potassium-exhausting impacts of corticosteroids, prompting an expanded gamble of hypokalemia. Customary checking of potassium levels and change of treatment might be fundamental.

5. Digoxin. Furosemide can modify the degrees of digoxin in the body, possibly expanding the gamble of digoxin poisonousness. Close observing of digoxin levels and fitting measurements changes are significant.

Drug-Regular Items

1. Licorice. Normal items containing licorice can lessen potassium levels in the body. When utilized simultaneously with furosemide, the gamble of hypokalemia might be expanded. Observing of potassium levels and changes in treatment might be essential.

2. St. John's Wort. St. John's Wort can incite liver proteins that utilize furosemide, possibly decreasing its viability. Alert is exhorted while utilizing St. John's Wort close by furosemide, and close checking of restorative reaction is essential.

Drug-Food

1. Grapefruit Juice. Grapefruit juice can slow down the digestion of furosemide, prompting expanded blood levels of the medicine. This can potentiate its belongings and increment the gamble of incidental effects. Try not to polish off

grapefruit or grapefruit juice while taking furosemide.

2. High-Salt Food varieties. Furosemide is a diuretic that assists with wiping out overabundance salt and liquid from the body. Eating high-salt food sources can neutralize the impacts of furosemide and diminish its adequacy. Following a decent, low-salt eating routine while taking furosemide is prudent.

Antagonistic Impacts

Furosemide is a diuretic medicine that is by and large very much endured and viable for overseeing liquid maintenance. Be that as it may, similar to any drug, it might possibly cause aftereffects and unfavorable responses. It is vital to know about these likely impacts to guarantee the protected utilization of furosemide. Here are a few normal incidental effects and unfriendly responses related with furosemide:

Normal Aftereffects

1. Expanded Pee. Furosemide is a diuretic that advances pee creation. Subsequently, expanded pee is a typical incidental effect. This impact is normal and generally not reason to worry.

Notwithstanding, on the off chance that it becomes extreme or is joined by other concerning side effects, counseling a medical care professional is significant.

2. Electrolyte Awkward nature. Furosemide can cause awkward nature in electrolyte levels, like low potassium (hypokalemia), low sodium (hyponatremia), and low magnesium (hypomagnesemia). These awkward nature can prompt side effects, for example, muscle cramps, shortcoming, unpredictable heartbeat, and exhaustion. Customary observing of electrolyte levels and fitting supplementation might be essential.

3. Unsteadiness and Wooziness. Furosemide can cause unsteadiness or wooziness, particularly while standing up rapidly. It is essential to rise gradually from a situated or lying position to limit the gamble of falls or injury.

4. Low Circulatory strain. Furosemide can bring down circulatory strain, prompting side effects like discombobulation, blacking out, or feeling dizzy. Checking of circulatory strain is significant, particularly in people with previous low pulse.

5. Migraine. A few people might encounter migraines as a symptom of furosemide. These cerebral pains are by and large gentle and determine all alone. If tenacious or extreme, counseling a medical services professional is fitting.

Antagonistic Responses

1. Hypersensitive Responses. Albeit uncommon, unfavorably susceptible responses to furosemide can happen. Side effects might incorporate skin rash, tingling, expanding, serious tipsiness, or trouble relaxing. On the off chance that any indications of an unfavorably susceptible response are capable, quick clinical consideration ought to be looked for.

2. Ototoxicity. Furosemide, especially when directed in high dosages or quickly imbued intravenously, can make harm the inward ear and lead to hearing misfortune or ringing in the ears (tinnitus). Brief announcing of any progressions in hearing is fundamental.

3. Extreme touchiness Responses. A few people might encounter extreme touchiness responses to furosemide, which can present as fever, skin rash, joint torment, or general discomfort. These

responses require clinical assessment and may require cessation of the drug.

4. Pancreatitis. Albeit intriguing, furosemide has been related with pancreatitis, an irritation of the pancreas. Side effects might incorporate extreme stomach agony, sickness, and heaving. Quick clinical consideration is fundamental on the off chance that pancreatitis is thought.

5. Erythema Multiforme (EM). Erythema multiforme is an uncommon skin problem described by the improvement of target-molded or "dead center" skin injuries. It is many times set off by an insusceptible reaction to contaminations or drugs, including furosemide. Side effects of EM might incorporate red, sketchy skin rash, target-formed sores with a red community and an encompassing ring, tingling or consuming sensation, and rankles or ulcerations in extreme cases.

6. Stevens-Johnson Disorder (SJS) and Harmful Epidermal Necrolysis (TEN). Stevens-Johnson disorder (SJS) and harmful epidermal necrolysis (TEN) are serious and possibly perilous skin conditions that can be brought about by specific prescriptions, including furosemide. They are

viewed as intriguing yet serious unfavorable responses. Side effects of SJS and TEN might incorporate difficult skin rash that spreads rapidly, skin rankling or stripping, mucous layer contribution (e.g., mouth, eyes, private parts), fever and influenza like side effects, and extreme skin torment and inconvenience.

7. Aplastic Pallor. Aplastic pallor is an uncommon however difficult condition described by a lessening in the creation of red platelets, white platelets, and platelets in the bone marrow. Albeit very intriguing, furosemide has been accounted for to be related with the improvement of aplastic paleness.

8. Agranulocytosis. Agranulocytosis is a serious condition portrayed by a critical decrease in the quantity of white platelets, explicitly granulocytes. Albeit rare, furosemide has been accounted for to cause agranulocytosis.

Organization Contemplations

Accessible Structures

Furosemide is accessible in the accompanying structures:

Tablets: 20 mg, 40 mg, 80 mg, 500 mg.

Oral arrangement (10 mg/mL — orange flavor, 8 mg/mL — pineapple — peach flavor): 8 mg/mL, 10 mg/mL.

Answer for infusion: 10 mg/mL.

Measurements for Children

Edema

PO (Youngsters): 1 - 4 mg/kg/portion 1 - twice/day.

IM, IV (Youngsters): 1 - 2 mg/kg/portion q 12 - 24 hr.

Measurements for Kids

Edema

PO (Kids >1 mo): 2 mg/kg as a solitary portion; might be expanded by 1-2 mg/kg q 6-8 hr (greatest portion = 6 mg/kg).

IM, IV (Kids): 1 - 2 mg/kg/portion q 6 - 12 hr persistent mixture — 0.05 mg/kg/hr, titrate to clinical impact.

Measurement for Grown-ups

Edema

PO (Grown-ups): 20 - 80 mg/day as a solitary portion at first, may rehash in 6-8 hr; may increment portion by 20-40 mg q 6-8 hr until wanted reaction. Support dosages might be given a few times every day (portions up to 2.5 g/day have been utilized in patients with HF or renal sickness). Hypertension — 40 two times day to day at first (when added to routine, decline portion of different anti-hypertensives by half); change further dosing in light of reaction; Hypercalcemia — 120 mg/day in 1 - 3 dosages.

IM, IV (Grown-ups): 20-40 mg, may rehash in 1-2 hr and inceased by 20 mg each 1 - 2 hr until reaction is gotten, support portion might be given q 6 - 12 hr; Consistent mixture — Bolus 0.1 mg/kg followed by 0.1 mg/kg/hr, twofold q 2 hr to a limit of 0.4 mg/kg/hr.

Hypertension

PO (Grown-ups): 40 two times every day at first (when added to routine, decline portion of different anti-hypertensives by half); change further dosing in view of reaction.

Pharmacokinetics

Understanding the pharmacokinetics of furosemide gives bits of knowledge into how the medicine is ingested, appropriated, utilized, and disposed of by the body. Here is an outline of the pharmacokinetic properties of furosemide:

1. Ingestion. Furosemide is all around ingested when taken orally, with roughly 60-70% of the portion arriving at foundational dissemination. The beginning of activity happens in no less than one hour after oral organization, with top impacts regularly saw inside 1-2 hours.

2. Appropriation. Furosemide has a generally enormous volume of dissemination, showing that it is circulated broadly all through the body. The prescription crosses the placenta and is found in bosom milk, so watchfulness ought to be practiced during pregnancy and breastfeeding.

3. Protein Restricting. Furosemide has a moderate level of protein restricting, basically to egg whites, a protein tracked down in the blood. Around 91-the vast majority of furosemide is bound to plasma

proteins. This limiting influences the dissemination and disposal of the medicine.

4. Digestion. Furosemide goes through negligible digestion in the liver. Most of the medication is discharged unaltered in the pee. Notwithstanding, a little part (under 10%) is used by hepatic chemicals to deliver latent metabolites.

5. End. Furosemide is essentially disposed of by the kidneys through both glomerular filtration and cylindrical discharge.

6. Half-life. The medicine has a generally short half-life, going from 30-an hour in people with ordinary renal capability. In people with disabled kidney capability, the half-life might be drawn out.

7. Measurements Changes. For people with hindered renal capability, dose changes might be important to guarantee protected and successful utilization of furosemide. It is vital to consider the person's creatinine freedom or assessed glomerular filtration rate (eGFR) while deciding the fitting dose.

8. Drug Associations. Furosemide can associate with different meds that influence renal capability or electrolyte balance. It is essential to audit the

singular's medicine profile and consider potential medication collaborations prior to starting furosemide treatment.

Nursing Contemplations for Furosemide

As a diuretic prescription, furosemide requires cautious nursing evaluation to guarantee protected and successful use.

Nursing Appraisal

Medical caretakers assume a crucial part in observing patients getting furosemide treatment. Here are key nursing evaluations and their reasoning while controlling furosemide:

1. Get an extensive clinical history, including any known sensitivities, kidney capability, liver sickness, heart conditions, electrolyte lopsided characteristics, and simultaneous drugs.

This appraisal recognizes possible contraindications, drug collaborations, and hazard factors for unfriendly impacts.

2. Routinely screen pulse, pulse, and respiratory rate. Furosemide's essential activity is to lessen liquid volume, prompting likely changes in circulatory strain and pulse.

Observing indispensable signs gives data about the drug's adequacy and guides suitable dosing changes.

3. Survey the patient's liquid equilibrium, including information and result estimations, day to day loads, and indications of liquid over-burden or parchedness.

Furosemide advances diuresis and can prompt liquid and electrolyte irregular characteristics. Checking liquid equilibrium decides the requirement for measurement changes and guides intercessions to keep up with satisfactory hydration.

4. Routinely screen electrolyte levels, especially potassium, sodium, and magnesium.

Furosemide can cause irregular characteristics in these electrolytes, prompting potential difficulties like heart arrhythmias or muscle shortcoming. Observing electrolyte levels distinguishes awkward nature and guides suitable mediations, like electrolyte supplementation.

5. Evaluate renal capability through research facility tests, for example, serum creatinine and assessed glomerular filtration rate (eGFR).

Furosemide is fundamentally killed by the kidneys, and hindered renal capability can influence drug leeway and increment the gamble of unfavorable impacts. Checking renal capability decides proper dosing and identifies any deteriorating of kidney capability.

6. Screen for indications of antagonistic responses, like hypersensitive responses (skin rash, tingling, trouble breathing), ototoxicity (changes in hearing or tinnitus), or serious skin responses (rankling, stripping).

Brief ID of antagonistic responses takes into account early intercession and avoidance of likely entanglements.

7. Give intensive patient schooling about furosemide, including measurement directions, possible secondary effects, the significance of consistence, and dietary contemplations (e.g., low-sodium diet).

Patient training advances understanding, adherence to the treatment plan, and self-administration of expected difficulties.

Furosemide Nursing Mediations

Medical caretakers' job in managing furosemide goes past evaluation. It likewise includes carrying out nursing mediations to guarantee the protected and powerful utilization of the prescription. Here are key nursing mediations and their reasoning while really focusing on patients getting furosemide treatment:

1. Direct furosemide as endorsed, guaranteeing the right measurements, course, and timing.

This mediation guarantees that patients get the expected remedial impacts of furosemide and keeps up with liquid equilibrium.

2. Archive the patient's liquid admission and result, everyday loads, and evaluate for indications of liquid over-burden or parchedness.

Furosemide advances diuresis, and checking liquid equilibrium decides the viability of the drug and guides changes in measurements and liquid administration.

3. Ceaselessly screen circulatory strain to survey the patient's reaction to furosemide treatment.

Furosemide's diuretic impact can bring down pulse, and observing recognizes hypotension or changes that might require dose changes or extra mediations.

4. Give exhaustive patient schooling about furosemide, including the reason for the medicine, dose guidelines, possible incidental effects, and the significance of adherence.

Enabling patients with information advances their dynamic support in their own consideration.

5. Teach patients about the signs and side effects of electrolyte irregular characteristics and when to look for clinical consideration.

Enabling patients with information advances their dynamic support in their own consideration.

6. Instruct patients on dietary changes, for example, following a low-sodium diet, if pertinent.

Sodium assumes a critical part in controlling liquid equilibrium in the body. At the point when sodium admission is high, it can prompt liquid maintenance and compound circumstances that require diuretic treatment. By following a low-sodium diet, patients can assist with keeping a more adjusted liquid status, which lines up with the objective of furosemide treatment.

7. Energize customary activity and weight the board to help liquid equilibrium and by and large cardiovascular wellbeing.

Customary activity can uphold liquid equilibrium by advancing flow and decreasing liquid maintenance. Active work further develops blood stream, which can help with the end of abundance liquid from the body. This synergistic impact of activity with furosemide can improve liquid equilibrium and diminish side effects of edema or liquid over-burden. Ordinary activity is known to have various cardiovascular advantages, including reinforcing the heart, further developing circulatory strain, and upgrading by and large cardiovascular capability.

8. Work together with the medical services group to give exhaustive consideration.

Furosemide treatment frequently includes overseeing complex ailments, like cardiovascular breakdown, kidney sickness, or hypertension. Teaming up with the medical services group takes into consideration a comprehensive way to deal with patient consideration, taking into account different parts of the patient's wellbeing, including clinical history, comorbidities, and therapy objectives. By cooperating, medical services experts can foster an extensive consideration plan that tends to the patient's extraordinary requirements and enhances therapy results.

9. Note any secondary effects or unfriendly responses of furosemide, like hypersensitive responses, ototoxicity, or serious skin responses.

Brief distinguishing proof and revealing of unfriendly impacts empower convenient intercessions to limit difficulties and work on quiet results.

10. Convey and team up with other medical services experts engaged with the patient's consideration, like doctors, drug specialists, and dietitians.

Sharing relevant data and looking for direction when required guarantee facilitated care and advance patient result

Patient Training and Instructing

Patient training and instructing are fundamental parts of care for patients getting furosemide. Instructing patients about their prescription assists them with grasping the reason, benefits, possible secondary effects, and important insurances. Here are key parts of patient instruction and educating, alongside their reasoning, for patients getting furosemide:

1. Clarify for the patient why furosemide has been recommended to them. Depict job as a diuretic drug takes out overabundance liquid from the body, lessening side effects like edema or windedness.

This understanding assists patients with perceiving the reason and advantages of accepting furosemide as recommended.

2. Give clear directions on the best way to take furosemide, including the suggested dose, recurrence, and timing.

Stress the significance of following the recommended timetable to keep up with steady restorative levels of the medicine in the body.

3. Teach patients about expected results of furosemide. Normal incidental effects might

incorporate expanded pee, electrolyte awkward nature, tipsiness, or migraine.

By monitoring possible aftereffects, patients can screen their side effects and immediately report any worries to their medical care supplier.

4. Make sense of the significance of keeping up with liquid and electrolyte balance while taking furosemide.

Furosemide works by advancing diuresis, which kills overabundance liquid from the body. Keeping up with liquid equilibrium is crucial for improve the drug's viability in decreasing side effects like edema, windedness, or liquid over-burden. By understanding the significance of liquid equilibrium, patients can effectively partake in dealing with their condition and upgrading treatment results.

5. Underline the need to follow any dietary changes, for example, a low-sodium diet, as endorsed.

A low-sodium diet supplements the prescription's activity by decreasing the general sodium consumption. Sodium adds to liquid maintenance, and by following a low-sodium diet, patients can upgrade the viability of furosemide in diminishing liquid development and dealing with their condition all the more really.

6. Talk about the significance of checking liquid admission and result, as well as indications of lack of hydration or electrolyte uneven characters.

Furosemide's diuretic impact can prompt expanded pee creation, possibly bringing about liquid misfortune. Making sense of the significance of checking liquid admission and result assists patients with perceiving the need to polish off a sufficient measure of liquids to forestall parchedness. Sufficient hydration guarantees ideal physical processes, upholds by and large prosperity, and forestalls confusions related with drying out.

7. Stress the meaning of accepting furosemide as endorsed and not skipping dosages.

Make sense of that predictable prescription adherence guarantees ideal helpful impacts and forestalls intricacies connected with liquid over-burden or deficient diuresis.

8. Illuminate patients about the requirement for standard observing, for example, circulatory strain

checks, lab tests (e.g., electrolyte levels, renal capability), and follow-up arrangements.

This checking permits medical services suppliers to survey the patient's reaction to furosemide, make any essential changes, and address any worries that might emerge.

9. Examine the significance of illuminating medical services suppliers pretty much all prescriptions, including non-prescription meds, enhancements, and natural items, to recognize possible collaborations with furosemide.

This information forestalls unfriendly impacts and guarantees the protected and viable utilization of prescriptions.

10. Instruct patients about security precautionary measures while taking furosemide. This incorporates rising gradually from a situated or lying position to limit unsteadiness, staying away from unnecessary sun openness, and perceiving indications of unfavorable responses, for example, skin rash or trouble relaxing.

11. Urge patients to look for sure fire clinical consideration on the off chance that they experience any disturbing side effects.

Furosemide, similar to any prescription, can cause unfavorable impacts in certain people. These impacts might incorporate extreme hypersensitive responses, changes in hearing, or skin responses. By empowering patients to speedily look for clinical consideration, medical services suppliers can evaluate the side effects and make suitable moves to address them. Early acknowledgment and intercession can forestall intricacies and advance patient security.

Assessment and Wanted Results

The ideal results in patients taking furosemide include:

1. Compelling Diuresis. Furosemide is a diuretic drug used to advance diuresis and decrease liquid maintenance. The ideal result is the successful end of overabundance liquid from the body, bringing about diminished edema, worked on breathing, and alleviation from side effects related with liquid over-burden.

2. Liquid Equilibrium. Accomplishing and keeping a decent liquid status is an ideal result. This includes forestalling liquid over-burden or drying out by changing the furosemide measurements or overseeing liquid admission. The patient ought to include stable liquid levels inside the objective reach, advancing by and large solace and prosperity.

3. Circulatory strain Control. Furosemide might be endorsed to oversee hypertension or decrease circulatory strain in patients with conditions like congestive cardiovascular breakdown. The ideal result is accomplishing and keeping up with target circulatory not entirely set in stone by the medical services supplier. Controlled circulatory strain decreases the gamble of intricacies related with hypertension and supports cardiovascular wellbeing.

4. Further developed Side effects. Furosemide is frequently endorsed to mitigate side effects related with liquid over-burden, like windedness, expanding, or weariness. The ideal result is a decrease in these side effects, prompting further developed practice resistance, improved personal

satisfaction, and generally speaking side effect help.

5. Electrolyte Equilibrium. Keeping a steady electrolyte balance is an ideal result. Furosemide can cause uneven characters in electrolytes, especially potassium, sodium, and magnesium. The objective is to keep electrolyte levels inside the ideal reach, forestalling inconveniences like cardiovascular arrhythmias or muscle shortcoming.

6. Medicine Adherence. Wanted results incorporate patients reliably sticking to the recommended furosemide routine. This includes accepting the drug as endorsed, following the suggested dose and recurrence. Adherence guarantees the drug's ideal remedial impacts and forestalls complexities connected with liquid over-burden or deficient diuresis.

7. Cooperation with the Medical care Group. An ideal result is successful cooperation and correspondence between the patient and the medical services group. This takes into consideration shared direction, open discourse, and extensive patient-focused care. Joint effort guarantees that the patient's interests are tended to,

treatment objectives are adjusted, and ideal results are accomplished.

What are IV Liquids?

Intravenous liquids (IV Liquids), otherwise called intravenous arrangements, are supplemental liquids utilized in intravenous treatment to reestablish or keep up with typical liquid volume and electrolyte balance when the oral course is unimaginable. IV liquid treatment is a proficient and successful approach to providing liquids straightforwardly into the intravascular liquid compartment, in supplanting electrolyte misfortunes, and in overseeing meds and blood items.

Sorts of IV Liquids

There are various sorts of IV liquids and various ways on the most proficient method to order them.

The most well-known method for sorting IV liquids depends on their constitution:

Isotonic. Isotonic IV arrangements that have similar grouping of solutes as blood plasma.

Hypotonic. Hypotonic arrangements have lesser centralization of solutes than plasma.

Hypertonic. Hypertonic arrangements have more prominent grouping of solutes than plasma.

IV arrangements can likewise be grouped in view of their motivation:

Supplement arrangements. May contain dextrose, glucose, and levulose to make up the sugar part - and water. Water is provided for liquid necessities and sugar for calories and energy. Supplement arrangements are helpful in forestalling lack of hydration and ketosis. Instances of supplement arrangements incorporate D5W, D5NSS.

Electrolyte arrangements. Contains fluctuating measures of cations and anions that are utilized to substitute liquid and electrolytes for clients with proceeding with misfortunes. Instances of electrolyte arrangements incorporate 0.9 NaCl, Ringer's Answer, and LRS.

Alkalinizing arrangements. Are directed to treat metabolic acidosis. Models: LRS.

Acidifying arrangements. Are utilized to check metabolic alkalosis. D51/2NS, 0.9 NaCl.

Volume expanders. Are arrangements used to build the blood volume after an extreme blood misfortune, or loss of plasma. Instances of volume expanders are dextran, human egg whites, and plasma.

Crystalloids

Crystalloid IV arrangements contain little atoms that stream effectively across semipermeable layers. They are sorted by their overall constitution according to plasma. There are three sorts: isotonic, hypotonic, and hypertonic.

Isotonic IV Liquids

Most IV liquids are isotonic, meaning, they have similar convergence of solutes as blood plasma. At the point when imbued, isotonic arrangements extend both the intracellular liquid and extracellular liquid spaces, similarly. Such liquids don't modify the osmolality of the vascular compartment. In fact, electrolyte arrangements are viewed as isotonic on the off chance that the absolute electrolyte content is roughly 310 mEq/L. Isotonic IV liquids have a complete osmolality near that of the ECF and don't make red platelets psychologist or swell.

Isotonic IV Liquids Cheat Sheet

Cheat sheet for Isotonic IV Liquids.

0.9% NaCl (Ordinary Saline Arrangement, NSS)

Typical saline arrangement (0.9% NaCl) or NSS, is a crystalloid isotonic IV liquid that contains water, sodium (154 mEq/L), and chloride (154 mEq/L). It has an osmolality of 308 mOsm/L and gives no calories. It is called typical saline arrangement on the grounds that the level of sodium chloride broke down in the arrangement is like the standard centralization of sodium and chloride in the intravascular space. Ordinary saline is the isotonic arrangement of decision for growing the extracellular liquid (ECF) volume since it doesn't enter the intracellular liquid (ICF). It is managed to address extracellular liquid volume shortfall since it stays inside the ECF.

Typical saline is the IV liquid utilized close by the organization of blood items. It is additionally used to supplant enormous sodium misfortunes like in consume wounds and injury. It ought not be utilized for cardiovascular breakdown, pneumonic edema, and renal impedance, or conditions that cause sodium maintenance as it might take a chance with liquid volume over-burden.

Dextrose 5% in Water (D5W)

D5W (dextrose 5% in water) is a crystalloid isotonic IV liquid with a serum osmolality of 252 mOsm/L. D5W is at first an isotonic arrangement and gives free water when dextrose is used (making it a hypotonic arrangement), growing the ECF and the ICF. It is managed to supply water and to address an expansion in serum osmolality. A liter of D5W gives less than 200 kcal and contains 50g of glucose. It ought not be utilized for liquid revival since hyperglycemia can result. It ought to likewise be kept away from to be utilized in clients in danger for expanded intracranial strain as it can cause cerebral edema.

Lactated Ringer's 5% Dextrose in Water (D5LRS)

Lactated Ringer's Answer (otherwise called Ringer's Lactate or Hartmann arrangement) is a crystalloid isotonic IV liquid intended to be the close physiological arrangement of adjusted electrolytes. It contains 130 mEq/L of sodium, 4 mEq/L of potassium, 3 mEq/L of calcium, and 109 mEq/L of chloride. It additionally contains bicarbonate forerunners to forestall acidosis. It doesn't give calories or magnesium and has restricted potassium substitution. It is the most physiologically versatile liquid on the grounds that its electrolyte content is most firmly connected with the synthesis of the body's blood serum and plasma.

Lactated Ringer's is utilized to address parchedness, sodium exhaustion, and supplant GI lot liquid misfortunes. It can likewise be utilized in liquid misfortunes because of consumes, fistula waste, and injury. It is the decision for first-line liquid revival for specific patients. It is frequently regulated to patients with metabolic acidosis.

Lactated Ringer's answer is utilized in the liver, which changes the lactate over completely to bicarbonate, consequently, it ought not be given to patients who can't use lactate (e.g., liver sickness, lactic acidosis). It ought to be utilized in alert for patients with cardiovascular breakdown and renal disappointment.

Ringer's Answer

Ringer's answer is another isotonic IV arrangement that has content like Lactated Ringer's Answer however doesn't contain lactate. Signs are no different for Lactated Ringer's except for without the contraindications connected with lactate.

Nursing Contemplations for Isotonic IV Arrangements

Coming up next are the general nursing mediations and contemplations while controlling isotonic arrangements:

Record pattern information. Prior to mixture, evaluate the patient's important bodily functions, edema status, lung sounds, and heart sounds. Keep checking during and after the implantation.

Notice for indications of liquid over-burden. Search for indications of hypervolemia like hypertension, bouncing heartbeat, aspiratory pops, dyspnea, windedness, fringe edema, jugular venous enlargement, and additional heart sounds.

Screen indications of proceeded with hypovolemia. Search for signs that demonstrate proceeded with hypovolemia, for example, diminished pee yield, unfortunate skin turgor, tachycardia, feeble heartbeat, and hypotension.

Forestall hypervolemia. Patients being treated for hypovolemia can rapidly foster liquid over-burden following quick or over imbuement of isotonic IV liquids.

Lift the top of the bed at 35 to 45 degrees. Except if contraindicated, position the client in semi-Fowler's situation.

Raise the patient's legs. Assuming that edema is available, hoist the legs of the patient to advance venous return.

Instruct patients and families. Train patients and families to perceive signs and side effects of liquid volume over-burden. Teach patients to advise their medical attendant assuming they experience difficulty breathing or notice any enlarging.

Close checking for patients with cardiovascular breakdown. Since isotonic liquids extend the intravascular space, patients with hypertension and cardiovascular breakdown ought to be painstakingly checked for indications of liquid over-burden.

Hypotonic IV Liquids

Hypotonic IV arrangements have a lower osmolality and contain less solutes than plasma.

They influence liquid movements from the ECF into the ICF to accomplish homeostasis, in this way, making cells expand and may try and burst. IV arrangements are viewed as hypotonic on the off chance that the absolute electrolyte content is under 250 mEq/L. Hypotonic IV liquids are generally used to give free water to discharge of body squanders, treat cell parchedness, and supplant the cell liquid.

0.45% Sodium Chloride (0.45% NaCl)

Sodium chloride 0.45% (1/2 NS), otherwise called half-strength ordinary saline, is a hypotonic IV arrangement utilized for supplanting water in patients who have hypovolemia with hypernatremia. Overabundance use might prompt hyponatremia because of the weakening of sodium, particularly in patients who are inclined to water maintenance. It has an osmolality of 154 mOsm/L and contains 77 mEq/L sodium and chloride. Hypotonic sodium arrangements are utilized to treat hypernatremia and other hyperosmolar conditions.

0.33% Sodium Chloride (0.33% NaCl)

Hypotonic IV Liquids and Arrangements Cheat Sheet

Cheat sheet for Hypotonic IV Liquids.

0.33% Sodium Chloride Arrangement is utilized to permit kidneys to hold the required measures of water and is regularly managed with dextrose to increment constitution. It ought to be utilized in alert for patients with cardiovascular breakdown and renal deficiency.

0.225% Sodium Chloride (0.225% NaCl)

0.225% Sodium Chloride Arrangement is in many cases utilized as an upkeep liquid for pediatric patients as it is the most hypotonic IV liquid accessible at 77 mOsm/L. Utilized along with dextrose.

2.5% Dextrose in Water (D2.5W)

Another hypotonic IV arrangement ordinarily utilized is 2.5% dextrose in water (D2.5W). This arrangement is utilized to treat lack of hydration and diminished the degrees of sodium and potassium. It ought not be regulated with blood items as it can cause hemolysis of red platelets.

Nursing Contemplations for Hypotonic IV Arrangements

Coming up next are the general nursing mediations and contemplations while managing hypotonic IV arrangements:

Record benchmark information. Prior to mixture, survey the patient's important bodily functions, edema status, lung sounds, and heart sounds. Keep observing during and after the mixture.

Try not to regulate in contraindicated conditions. Hypotonic arrangements might intensify existing hypovolemia and hypotension causing cardiovascular breakdown. Stay away from use in patients with liver sickness, injury, or consumes.

Risk for expanded intracranial strain (IICP). Ought not be given to patients with risk for IICP as the liquid shift might cause cerebral edema (recollect: hypotonic arrangements make cells enlarge).

Screen for signs of liquid volume deficiency. Signs and side effects remember disarray for more established grown-ups. Educate patients to illuminate the medical caretaker assuming that they feel dazed.

Cautioning on inordinate mixture. Inordinate mixture of hypotonic IV liquids can prompt intravascular liquid exhaustion, diminished circulatory strain, cell edema, and cell harm.

Try not to manage alongside blood items. Most hypotonic arrangements can cause hemolysis of red platelets particularly during fast implantation of the arrangement.

Hypertonic IV Liquids

Hypertonic IV arrangements have a more prominent convergence of solutes (375 mEq/L and more noteworthy) than plasma and prompt liquids to move out of the cells and into the ECF to standardize the grouping of particles between two compartments. This impact makes cells contract and may upset their capability. They are otherwise called volume expanders as they coax water out of the intracellular space, expanding extracellular liquid volume.

Hypertonic IV Liquids and Arrangements Cheat Sheet

Cheat sheet for Hypertonic IV Liquids.

Hypertonic Sodium Chloride IV Liquids

Hypertonic sodium chloride arrangements contain a higher grouping of sodium and chloride than ordinarily contained in plasma. Implantation of hypertonic sodium chloride arrangement shifts liquids from the intracellular space into the intravascular and interstitial spaces. Hypertonic sodium chloride IV arrangements are accessible in the accompanying structures and qualities:

3% sodium chloride (3% NaCl) containing 513 mEq/L of sodium and chloride with an osmolality of 1030 mOsm/L.

5% sodium chloride (5% NaCl) containing 855 mEq/L of sodium and chloride with an osmolality of 1710 mOsm/L.

Hypertonic sodium chloride arrangements are utilized in the intense therapy of sodium lack (extreme hyponatremia) and ought to be utilized exclusively in basic circumstances to treat hyponatremia. They should be imbued at an extremely low rate to stay away from the gamble of over-burden and pneumonic edema. Whenever controlled in huge amounts and quickly, they might cause an extracellular volume abundance and encourage circulatory over-burden and lack of hydration. In this manner, they ought to be managed carefully and generally just when the serum osmolality has diminished to basically low levels. A few patients might require diuretic treatment to aid liquid discharge. It is likewise utilized in patients with cerebral edema.

Hypertonic Dextrose Arrangements

Isotonic arrangements that contain 5% dextrose (e.g., D5NSS, D5LRS) are marginally hypertonic since they surpass the absolute osmolality of the ECF. In any case, dextrose is immediately utilized and just the isotonic arrangement remains. Consequently, any impact on the ICF is transitory. Hypertonic dextrose arrangements are utilized to give kilocalories to the patient for the time being. Higher groupings of dextrose (i.e., D50W) are solid hypertonic arrangements and should be directed into focal veins so they can be weakened by quick blood stream.

Dextrose 10% in Water (D10W)

Dextrose 10% in Water (D10W) is a hypertonic IV arrangement utilized in the treatment of ketosis of starvation and gives calories (380 kcal/L), free water, and no electrolytes. It ought to be directed utilizing a focal line in the event that conceivable and ought not be mixed involving similar line as blood items as it can cause RBC hemolysis.

Dextrose 20% in Water (D20W)

Dextrose 20% in Water (D20W) is hypertonic IV arrangement an osmotic diuretic that makes liquid movements between different compartments advance diuresis.

Dextrose half in Water (D50W)

Another hypertonic IV arrangement utilized ordinarily is Dextrose half in Water (D50W) which is utilized to treat extreme hypoglycemia and is regulated quickly by means of IV bolus.

Nursing Contemplations for Hypertonic IV Liquids

Coming up next are the general nursing mediations and contemplations while overseeing hypertonic IV arrangements:

Record gauge information. Prior to mixture, evaluate the patient's important bodily functions, edema status, lung sounds, and heart sounds. Keep observing during and after the mixture.

Watch for indications of hypervolemia. Since hypertonic arrangements move liquid from the ICF to the ECF, they increment the extracellular liquid volume and builds the gamble for hypervolemia. Search for indications of enlarging in arms, legs, face, windedness, hypertension, and uneasiness in the body (e.g., migraine, squeezing).

Screen and notice the patient during organization. Hypertonic arrangements ought to be controlled exclusively in high sharpness regions with steady nursing reconnaissance for expected confusions.

Check request. Remedy for hypertonic arrangements ought to express the particular hypertonic liquid to be implanted, the complete volume to be imbued, the mixture rate and the timeframe to proceed with the implantation.

Survey wellbeing history. Patients with kidney or coronary illness and the individuals who are got dried out shouldn't get hypertonic IV liquids. These arrangements can influence renal filtration instruments and can undoubtedly cause hypervolemia to patients with renal or heart issues.

Forestall liquid over-burden. Guarantee that organization of hypertonic liquids doesn't accelerate liquid volume overabundance or over-burden.

Try not to manage incidentally. Hypertonic arrangements can make disturbance and harm the vein and ought to be controlled through a focal vascular access gadget embedded into a focal vein.

Screen blood glucose intently. Quick imbuement of hypertonic dextrose arrangements can cause hyperglycemia. Use with alert for patients with diabetes mellitus.

Colloids

Colloids contain huge particles that don't go through semipermeable films. Colloids are IV liquids that contain solutes of high sub-atomic weight, actually, they are hypertonic arrangements, which when implanted, apply an osmotic draw of liquids from interstitial and extracellular spaces. They are helpful for growing the intravascular volume and raising pulse. Colloids are demonstrated for patients in malnourished states and patients who can't endure enormous implantations of liquid.

Human Egg whites

Human egg whites is an answer gotten from plasma. It has two qualities: 5% egg whites and 25% egg whites. 5% Egg whites is an answer gotten from plasma and is a normally used colloid arrangement. It is utilized to build the flowing volume and reestablish protein levels in conditions like consumes, pancreatitis, and plasma misfortune through injury. 25% Egg whites is utilized along with sodium and water limitation to decrease unreasonable edema. They are viewed as blood bonding items and utilizations similar conventions and nursing safety measures while regulating egg whites.

The utilization of egg whites is contraindicated in patients with the accompanying circumstances: extreme weakness, cardiovascular breakdown, or known aversion to egg whites. Furthermore, angiotensin-changing over protein inhibitors ought to be kept for somewhere around 24 hours prior to managing egg whites on account of the gamble of abnormal responses, like hypotension and flushing.

Dextrans

Dextrans are polysaccharides that go about as colloids. They are accessible in two kinds: low-atomic weight dextrans (LMWD) and high-sub-atomic weight dextrans (HMWD). They are accessible in one or the other saline or glucose arrangements. Dextran obstructs blood crossmatching, so draw the patient's blood prior to managing dextran, assuming that crossmatching is expected.

Low-sub-atomic weight Dextrans (LMWD)

LMWD contains polysaccharide particles that act like colloids with a typical atomic load of 40,000 (Dextran 40). LMWD is utilized to work on the microcirculation in patients with unfortunate fringe course. They contain no electrolytes and are utilized to treat shock connected with vascular volume misfortune (e.g., consumes, discharge, injury, or medical procedure). On specific surgeries, LMWDs are utilized to forestall venous thromboembolism. They are contraindicated in patients with thrombocytopenia, hypofibrinogenemia, and extreme touchiness to dextran.

High-sub-atomic weight Dextrans (HMWD)

HMWD contains polysaccharide particles with a typical atomic load of 70,000 (Dextran 70) or 75,000 (Dextran 75). HMWD utilized for patients with hypovolemia and hypotension. They are contraindicated in patients with hemorrhagic shock.

Etherified Starch

These arrangements are gotten from starch and are utilized to increment intravascular liquid however can disrupt typical coagulation. Models incorporate EloHAES,

Gelatin

Gelatins have lower sub-atomic load than dextrans and consequently stay in the dissemination for a more limited timeframe.

Plasma Protein Division (PPF)

Plasma Protein Division is an answer that is likewise ready from plasma, and like egg whites, is warmed before implantation. It is prescribed to inject gradually to increment circling volume.

Nursing Contemplations for Colloid IV Arrangements

Coming up next are the general nursing mediations and contemplations while controlling colloid IV arrangements:

Survey sensitivity history. Most colloids can cause hypersensitive responses, albeit intriguing, so take a cautious sensitivity history, asking explicitly on the off chance that they've at any point had a response to an IV implantation.

Utilize a huge drag needle (18-check). A bigger needle is required while controlling colloid arrangements.

Archive pattern information. Prior to implantation, evaluate the patient's important bodily functions, edema status, lung sounds, and heart sounds. Keep observing during and after the implantation.

Screen the patient's reaction. Screen admission and result intently for indications of hypervolemia, hypertension, dyspnea, snaps in the lungs, and edema.

Screen coagulation lists. Colloid arrangements can slow down platelet capability and increment draining times, so screen the patient's coagulation files.

Gabapentin is a drug generally recommended to treat different circumstances, including epilepsy, neuropathic torment, and fretful legs condition. This guide intends to teach patients about significant contemplations, including dose directions, expected aftereffects, and precautionary measures, to guarantee protected and compelling utilization of gabapentin.

What is Gabapentin?

Gabapentin is an anticonvulsant prescription that is basically used to treat epilepsy. It is likewise recommended for different circumstances, for example, neuropathic torment, anxious legs disorder, and hot glimmers. It works by influencing the action of specific synapses in the cerebrum, explicitly focusing on calcium channels. Gabapentin works by influencing the movement of specific synapses in the mind, explicitly focusing on calcium channels. By regulating these channels, it assists with lessening the extreme electrical movement in the mind that can prompt seizures in people with epilepsy. Gabapentin has shown viability in alleviating neuropathic torment, which is brought about by harm or brokenness of the nerves. It is accepted to work by hindering the transmission of agony signals in the sensory system. While gabapentin is by and large very much endured, it might cause incidental effects like sluggishness, tipsiness, and coordination issues. It can likewise cooperate with specific meds, so illuminating the medical services supplier pretty much all ongoing drugs and ailments prior to beginning treatment is significant.

Conventional Name

gabapentin

Brand Names

Here are some normal brand names under which gabapentin is promoted:

- Neurontin
- Gralise
- Horizant
- Gabarone
- Fanatrex
- Gabapin
- Gabapentin Intas
- Gabapentin Sandoz
- Gabapentin Teva
- Neurontin

Drug Arrangement of Gabapentin

The medication arrangement of gabapentin is:

Remedial Class

- pain relieving assistants
- anticonvulsant
- state of mind stabilizers

Signs and Remedial Impacts

Gabapentin is demonstrated for the treatment of different circumstances, including:

1. Epilepsy. It is ordinarily endorsed as an adjunctive treatment for the treatment of halfway seizures in grown-ups and youngsters.

2. Neuropathic torment. Gabapentin is utilized to lighten neuropathic torment, which can result from conditions like diabetic neuropathy, post-herpetic neuralgia (nerve torment following shingles), and fringe neuropathy.

3. Anxious Legs Condition (RLS). It very well may be recommended to diminish the awkward sensations and desire to move the legs that describe RLS.

4. Fibromyalgia. Gabapentin might be utilized to assist with dealing with the aggravation related with fibromyalgia, a persistent issue portrayed by

far and wide outer muscle agony, exhaustion, and delicacy.

5. Hot glimmers. It has been viewed as successful in diminishing the recurrence and seriousness of hot blazes experienced by menopausal ladies.

6. Off-mark utilizes. Gabapentin might be endorsed off-mark for conditions, for example, nervousness issues, bipolar confusion, headache avoidance, and liquor withdrawal side effects.

Component of Activity

The instrument of activity isn't known, yet managing different mechanisms is accepted. Gabapentin fundamentally acts by restricting to a particular subunit of voltage-gated calcium directs in the focal sensory system. This limiting decreases the arrival of a few synapses, including glutamate, norepinephrine, and substance P, which are engaged with the transmission of torment signals.

Likewise, gabapentin expands the blend and arrival of gamma-aminobutyric corrosive (GABA), an inhibitory synapse that controls neuronal sensitivity. By upgrading GABA levels, gabapentin advances a quieting impact on overactive nerve flags and may add to its antiepileptic and anxiolytic properties.

Moreover, gabapentin has been displayed to tweak specific synapse receptors, for example, the alpha-2-delta subunit of voltage-gated calcium channels. This balance might additionally add to its pain relieving and anticonvulsant impacts.

Precautionary measures and Contraindications

Prior to taking gabapentin, it is vital to know about the accompanying precautionary measures and contraindications:

1. Sensitivity. People with a known sensitivity or extreme touchiness to gabapentin ought to keep away from its utilization.

2. Kidney issues. Gabapentin is essentially disposed of from the body through the kidneys. Subsequently, people with impeded kidney capability or those going through dialysis might require measurement changes or close observing.

3. Psychological wellness issues. Gabapentin has been related with an expanded gamble of self-destructive contemplations and ways of behaving.

People with a background marked by discouragement, mind-set issues, or self-destructive inclinations ought to be firmly checked while taking gabapentin.

4. Substance misuse. Gabapentin has the potential for misuse and reliance, especially when joined with different substances. People with a background marked by substance misuse or habit ought to practice alert and be firmly checked while taking gabapentin.

5. Pregnancy and breastfeeding. The utilization of gabapentin during pregnancy or breastfeeding ought to be examined with a medical care proficient. It might represent specific dangers to the creating baby or nursing newborn child.

6. Communications with different prescriptions. Gabapentin might collaborate with specific drugs, for example, narcotics or focal sensory system depressants, prompting expanded sedation and respiratory despondency. It is significant to illuminate the medical services supplier pretty much all ongoing prescriptions, including non-prescription medications and home grown supplements, prior to beginning gabapentin.

7. Driving and working apparatus. Gabapentin might cause sleepiness, unsteadiness, and coordination issues. It is vital to try not to drive or working apparatus until the singular knows what the prescription means for them.

Drug Collaborations

Gabapentin can interface with different drugs, regular items, and food. It is vital to know about these potential medication associations.

Drug-Medication

Gabapentin might possibly connect with a few different prescriptions, and it is essential to know about these medication drug communications. Here are a few models:

1. Narcotics. Joining gabapentin with narcotics, like morphine or oxycodone, can build the gamble of focal sensory system melancholy, respiratory gloom, and sedation. Close checking is vital, and dose changes might be required.

2. CNS depressants. Gabapentin can improve the soothing impacts of other focal sensory system depressants, including benzodiazepines, narcotics,

sedatives, and liquor. The blend can prompt unreasonable sluggishness, unsteadiness, and disabled coordination. Wariness and dose changes might be fundamental.

3. Stomach settling agents. Taking gabapentin with aluminum or magnesium-containing stomach settling agents can diminish the ingestion of gabapentin from the gastrointestinal lot. To stay away from this association, isolating the organization of gabapentin and stomach settling agents by something like 2 hours is suggested.

4. Naproxen. Consolidating gabapentin with naproxen, a nonsteroidal mitigating drug (NSAID), can expand the gamble of kidney harm. Close checking of kidney capability is exhorted while utilizing these drugs together.

5. Diuretics: A few diuretics, like hydrochlorothiazide, can expand the disposal of gabapentin from the body, possibly lessening its viability. Measurement changes might be fundamental in such cases.

6. Morphine. Gabapentin might expand the degrees of morphine in the body, prompting an expanded gamble of secondary effects. Close observing is

significant in the event that these prescriptions are utilized associatively.

Drug-Regular Items

Gabapentin might collaborate with specific regular items, and it is essential to know about these likely connections. Here are a few models:

1. St. John's Wort. St. John's Wort is a natural enhancement utilized for state of mind problems. It can actuate liver catalysts, which might diminish the degrees of gabapentin in the body, possibly lessening its adequacy. Close observing and measurements changes might be vital assuming these are utilized together.

2. Melatonin. Melatonin is a characteristic chemical that controls rest wake cycles. Joining gabapentin with melatonin might expand the soothing impacts and cause over the top sleepiness. Alert is prompted while utilizing these together, particularly while driving or working apparatus.

3. Home grown narcotics. Certain home grown narcotics, for example, valerian root and kava, may upgrade the calming impacts of gabapentin, prompting expanded tiredness and disabled coordination. Alert is encouraged, and changing

the measurement or timing of administration might be essential.

4. Ginkgo Biloba. Ginkgo biloba is a natural enhancement normally utilized for memory upgrade. There have been reports of seizures happening in people taking gabapentin and ginkgo biloba simultaneously. Close checking is significant if utilizing these together.

5. Pot. Pot items, especially those containing tetrahydrocannabinol (THC), may build the calming impacts of gabapentin. Alert is exhorted while consolidating these substances, as it might bring about inordinate sluggishness and weakened mental capability.

Drug-Food

With regards to food connections, gabapentin by and large has no critical collaborations with explicit food varieties. Nonetheless, there are a couple of variables connected with food that ought to be thought about while taking gabapentin:

1. Ingestion. Gabapentin is better consumed by the body when taken with food. While it tends to be taken regardless of food, taking it with a dinner

might upgrade its retention and increment its viability.

2. Timing. In the event that the doctor has endorsed gabapentin to be taken on various occasions a day, keeping a steady timetable with respect to food intake is significant. Taking it with feasts or snacks at standard spans might be considered to guarantee a consistent degree of drug in the framework.

Unfavorable Impacts

Gabapentin, similar to any prescription, might possibly cause secondary effects and unfriendly responses in certain people. Not every person will encounter these impacts, and the seriousness and recurrence of incidental effects can differ. Here are a few normal incidental effects related with gabapentin:

1. Sluggishness or tipsiness. Gabapentin can cause sluggishness or tipsiness, particularly while at first taking it or when the dose is expanded. Vital to keep away from exercises require mental sharpness, like driving or working hardware.

2. Weakness. A few people might encounter expanded weakness or sleepiness while taking gabapentin.

3. Coordination troubles. Gabapentin can influence coordination and equilibrium in certain individuals, prompting troubles in developments.

4. Sickness and spewing. These gastrointestinal side effects can happen, especially toward the start of treatment, yet they as a rule improve with time.

5. Weight gain. A few people might encounter weight gain while taking gabapentin. It is vital to keep a sound way of life and examine any worries with the medical care supplier.

6. Temperament changes. In uncommon cases, gabapentin might cause temperament changes, including expanded tension or despondency.

7. Unfavorably susceptible responses. While interesting, a few people might encounter hypersensitive responses to gabapentin, like skin rash, tingling, enlarging, or trouble relaxing.

Organization Contemplations

Accessible Structures

Gabapentin is accessible in the accompanying structures:

Cases: 100 mg, 300 mg, 400 mg.

Tablets: 600 mg, 800 mg.

Expanded discharge tablets (Horizant): 600 mg.

Supported discharge tablets (Gralise): 300 mg, 600 mg.

Oral arrangement (cool strawberry anise flavor): 250 mg/5 mL.

Dose for Kids

Epilepsy

PO (Youngsters >12 yr): 300 mg multiple times every day at first. Titration might be gone on until wanted (range is 900 - 1800 mg/day in 3 partitioned dosages; portions ought not be in excess of 12 hr separated). Portions up to 2400 - 3600 mg/day have been very much endured.

PO (Youngsters ≥5 - 12 yr): 10 - 15 mg/kg/day in 3 isolated dosages at first titrated vertical more than 3 days to 25-35 mg/kg/day in 3 partitioned dosages; dose span shouldn't surpass 12 hrs. (portions up to 50 mg/kg/day have been utilized).

PO (Kids 3 - 4 yrs): 10 - 15 mg/kg/day in 3 isolated portions at first titrated vertical north of 3 days to 40 mg/kg/day in 3 partitioned dosages; measurement span shouldn't surpass 12 hrs. (dosages up to 50 mg/kg/day have been utilized).

Renal Hindrance

PO (Youngsters >12 yr): CCr 30 - 59 mL/min — 200-700 mg two times day to day; CCr 15-29 mL/min — 200 - 700 mg once day to day; CCr 15 mL/min — 100 - 300 mg once every day; CCr <15 mL/min — Decrease day to day portion in relation to CCr.

Neuropathic Torment (unlabeled use)

PO (Youngsters): 5 mg/kg/portion at sleep time at first, then increment to 5 mg/kg BID on day 2 and 5mg/kg TID on day 3. Titrate to impact up to 8 - 35 mg/kg/day in 3 partitioned portions.

Dose for Grown-ups

Epilepsy

PO (Grown-ups): 300 mg multiple times every day at first. Titration might be gone on until wanted (range is 900 - 1800 mg/day in 3 separated dosages; portions ought not be in excess of 12 hr separated). Portions up to 2400 - 3600 mg/day have been very much endured.

Renal Impedance

PO (Grown-ups): CCr 30 - 59 mL/min — 200-700 mg two times day to day; CCr 15-29 mL/min — 200 - 700 mg once day to day; CCr 15 mL/min — 100 - 300 mg once every day; CCr <15 mL/min — Lessen day to day portion with respect to CCr.

PO (Grown-ups): CCr 30 - 59 mL/min — 200 - 700 mg two times day to day (quick delivery); 600 - 1800 mg once day to day (supported discharge [Gralise]); 300 mg once day to day in the first part of the day on days 1 - 3, then 300 mg two times day to day from there on (may increment to 600 mg two times day to day, depending on the situation) (expanded discharge [Horizant]); CCr 15 - 29 mL/min — 200 - 700 mg once day to day (prompt delivery); supported discharge [Gralise] not suggested; 300 mg in that frame of mind on days 1 and 3, then 300 mg once day to day in the first part of the day from there on (may increment to 300 mg two times day to day, depending on the situation) (broadened discharge [Horizant]); CCr 15 mL/min — 100 - 300 mg once day to day (prompt delivery); supported discharge [Gralise] not suggested; CCr ——————————15 mL/min — decline day to day portion in relation to CCr (im-intercede discharge); supported discharge [Gralise] not suggested; 300 mg each and every day toward the beginning of the day (may increment to 300 mg once day to day toward the beginning of the day, depending on the situation) (broadened discharge [Horizant]); CCr <15 mL/min (on hemodialysis) — 300 mg after every dialysis meeting (may increment to 600 mg after every dialysis meetings, as needed)(extended-discharge [Horizant]).

(Grown-ups): CCr 30 - 59 mL/min — 300 mg once day to day at 5 PM; may increment to 600 mg once day to day at 5 PM on a case by case basis; CCr 15-29 mL/min — 300 mg once day to day at 5 PM; CCr <15 mL/min — 300 mg each and every other day; CCr <15 mL/min (on hemodialysis) — Not suggested.

Postherpetic Neuralgia

PO (Grown-ups): Prompt delivery — 300 mg once every mday on first day, then, at that point, 300 mg twice day to day on second day, then, at that point, 300 mg multiple times/day on day 3, may then be titrated vertical depending on the situation up to 600 mg multiple times/day; Supported discharge (Gralise) — 300 mg once day to day on first day, then, at that point, 600 mg once day to day on second day, then 900 mg once day to day on days 3 - 6, then 1200 mg once day to day on days 7 - 10, then 1500 mg once day to day on days 11 - 14, then 1800 mg once day to day from there on; Broadened discharge (Horizant) — 600 mg once day to day in the first part of the day on days 1 - 3, then 600 mg two times day to day from that point.

Fretful Legs Disorder

PO (Grown-ups): Expanded discharge (Horizant) — 600 mg once day to day at 5 PM.

Neuropathic Agony (unlabeled use)

PO (Grown-ups): 100 mg multiple times day to day at first. Titrate week after week by 300 mg/day up to 900 - 2400 mg/day (most extreme: 3600 mg/day).

Pharmacokinetics

Understanding the pharmacokinetics of gabapentin assists medical care experts with deciding fitting doses and consider potential medication cooperations or changes in view of renal capability.

1. Retention. Gabapentin is very much assimilated after oral organization, with top plasma fixations commonly arrived at inside 2 to 3 hours. Food may somewhat postpone its ingestion.

2. Bioavailability. The bioavailability of gabapentin is around 60%, intending that around 60% of the portion taken arrives at the fundamental flow.

3. Protein restricting. Gabapentin has negligible plasma protein restricting, with under 3% bound to proteins in the blood.

4. Dissemination. Gabapentin is generally circulated all through the body, including crossing the blood-mind boundary. It has a somewhat huge volume of circulation, showing broad tissue dispersion.

5. Digestion. Gabapentin goes through negligible digestion in the liver. It isn't widely utilized by cytochrome P450 chemicals and doesn't altogether repress or incite these catalysts.

6. End. Gabapentin is essentially wiped out unaltered through the kidneys.

7. Half-life. It has an end half-existence of roughly 5 to 7 hours in people with typical kidney capability. In any case, in people with disabled renal capability, the disposal half-life might be drawn out.

8. Renal change. Portion changes might be fundamental for people with weakened renal capability to stay away from gabapentin gathering. The specific change relies upon the person's renal capability and ought not entirely set in stone by a medical services proficient.

Nursing Contemplations for Gabapentin

While directing or really focusing on patients taking gabapentin, medical attendants ought to think about a few significant variables.

Nursing Appraisal

1. Survey the patient's clinical history, including any known sensitivities, past unfriendly responses to gabapentin or comparative drugs, and applicable ailments.

This data distinguishes possible contraindications or safeguards for gabapentin use.

2. Assess the patient's ongoing side effects, for example, seizures, nerve torment, or anxious legs condition.

To decide the suitability of gabapentin as a treatment choice and to lay out standard information for evaluating treatment viability.

3. Audit the patient's medicine history, including remedy and non-prescription meds, to distinguish any potential medication connections with gabapentin.

This appraisal forestalls antagonistic medication responses and guarantees safe drug organization.

4. Survey the patient's renal capability through research facility tests, for example, serum creatinine and assessed glomerular filtration rate (eGFR).

Gabapentin is essentially disposed of through the kidneys, so debilitated renal capability might require dose changes in accordance with forestall drug collection and related secondary effects.

5. Play out a neurological evaluation, including appraisal of tangible and engine capability, reflexes, and coordination.

This evaluation lays out a gauge for correlation and recognizes any expected neurological symptoms of gabapentin.

6. Assess the patient's aggravation level, area, force, and quality.

Gabapentin is frequently endorsed for neuropathic torment, so checking torment levels and reaction to treatment is urgent for evaluating the adequacy of the drug.

7. Evaluate the patient's emotional wellness status, including temperament, uneasiness levels, and any set of experiences of sorrow or self-destructive ideation.

Gabapentin might cause temperament changes or increment the gamble of self-destructive considerations, so checking psychological well-being is significant for early recognition and intercession.

8. Screen and survey for likely results of gabapentin, like sluggishness, dazedness, exhaustion, or gastrointestinal side effects.

Surveying for these unfavorable impacts guarantees patient security and prosperity.

9. Assess the's comprehension patient might interpret gabapentin, including its motivation, measurement routine, expected aftereffects, and the significance of prescription adherence.

Evaluating the patient's consistence and instructive necessities considers suitable help and support of medicine directions.

.

Gabapentin Nursing Mediations

1. Direct gabapentin as indicated by the endorsed measurements and timetable.

This guarantees that the patient gets the proper portion of prescription brilliantly, advancing helpful impacts.

2. Give exhaustive training to the patient about gabapentin, including its motivation, anticipated benefits, expected secondary effects, and legitimate organization strategies.

Instruction engages the patient to pursue informed choices, stick to the medicine routine, and perceive and report any antagonistic impacts.

3. Teach the patient about possible symptoms of gabapentin, like sluggishness, wooziness, or coordination hardships.

By giving data about expected incidental effects, patients can arrive at informed conclusions about their treatment. They can gauge the advantages of gabapentin against the likely dangers and conclude whether the medicine is reasonable for them.

4. Encourage the patient to practice alert while participating in exercises that require sharpness, like driving or working apparatus.

Incidental effects like sleepiness, dazedness, or coordination troubles can present dangers. Patients should know about these possible impacts to avoid potential risk.

5. Advance the utilization of security measures, like handrails or assistive gadgets.

To forestall falls.

6. Work together with the medical services group to foster a thorough agony the executives plan.

Torment the board requires a comprehensive methodology that thinks about the patient's remarkable necessities, clinical history, and current condition. By teaming up with the medical services group, including doctors, attendants, drug specialists, and different subject matter experts, an extensive aggravation the board plan can be formed that considers different elements adding to the patient's aggravation, like the fundamental condition, seriousness of torment, and expected communications with different prescriptions.

7. Change torment the board intercessions as the need might arise.

To guarantee ideal agony control.

8. Record any progressions or upgrades in side effects, as well as any new or demolishing side effects.

For ideal intercession or change of the treatment plan.

9. Offer close to home help and guiding to patients who might encounter state of mind changes, uneasiness, or other psychological well-being impacts related with gabapentin.

Temperament changes, nervousness, or other emotional well-being impacts can fundamentally influence a patient's prosperity and personal satisfaction. By offering profound help and directing, medical care suppliers can assist patients with adapting with these impacts, diminish trouble, and work on their in general emotional well-being.

10. Offer assets or reference to emotional well-being experts if necessary.

A few patients might encounter extreme or industrious psychological well-being side effects while taking gabapentin, like serious melancholy, self-destructive considerations, or huge uneasiness. These side effects might require specific emotional well-being intercessions that stretch out past the extent of the essential medical services supplier.

Patient Schooling and Instructing

1. Make sense of the reason for gabapentin, for example, overseeing seizures, nerve torment, or different circumstances.

Understanding the reason why they are taking the drug assists patients with perceiving the expected advantages and spurs adherence to the endorsed treatment plan.

2. Give clear directions on the legitimate measurements and timetable for taking gabapentin.

Accepting the prescription as recommended guarantees reliable levels in the body, enhancing its viability and limiting the gamble of missed or twofold portions.

3. Stress the significance of adherence to the endorsed routine and make sense of the likely outcomes of missed portions or conflicting use.

Predictable utilization of gabapentin is important to keep up with restorative levels in the body and accomplish the ideal treatment results.

4. Instruct patients about possible results of gabapentin, like tiredness, unsteadiness, or gastrointestinal side effects.

Monitoring potential secondary effects helps patients perceive and ascribe these side effects to the drug, advancing early revealing and fitting administration.

5. Examine wellbeing precautionary measures connected with gabapentin, for example, keeping

away from exercises that require sharpness or utilizing alert while driving or working apparatus because of possible sluggishness or unsteadiness.

Patient getting it and adherence to somewhere safe and secure precautionary measures decrease the gamble of mishaps or falls, advancing generally security and prosperity.

6. Make sense of a particular food or medication co-operations that might influence gabapentin's retention or viability, for example, taking it regardless of food and staying away from liquor.

Appropriate organization and aversion of communications upgrade the ingestion and remedial impacts of gabapentin.

7. Feature the significance of going to follow-up meetings with medical care suppliers to screen the viability of gabapentin, survey for aftereffects, and make any essential acclimations to the therapy plan.

Normal follow-up guarantees that the treatment stays proper and successful, and takes into consideration ideal intercessions or alterations if necessary.

8. Train patients to report any strange or extreme secondary effects or antagonistic responses to their medical services supplier quickly.

Opportune detailing of unfavorable responses works with early intercession, limits possible mischief, and takes into account proper administration.

9. Give directions on the most proficient method to store gabapentin appropriately, for example, at room temperature, away from dampness and intensity.

Legitimate capacity guarantees drug respectability and adequacy.

10. Urge patients to clarify pressing issues, look for explanation, or express worries in regards to gabapentin.

Open correspondence and patient commitment advance grasping, upgrade treatment adherence, and take into account complete patient-focused care.

Assessment and Wanted Results

While assessing the utilization of gabapentin, medical services suppliers survey the patient's reaction to therapy and measure the accomplishment of wanted results. Here are a few assessment measures and wanted results for gabapentin:

1. Decrease in seizures. For patients endorsed gabapentin to oversee seizures, the ideal result is a decrease in the recurrence, length, or seriousness of seizures. Assessment includes following the number and power of seizures after some time and surveying any progressions or upgrades.

2. Help with discomfort. In situations where gabapentin is utilized for the administration of nerve torment, the ideal result is a decrease in torment power or further developed torment control. Assessment incorporates evaluating the patient's aggravation levels, utilizing torment scales or abstract reports, and observing changes in torment discernment and usefulness.

3. Further developed rest. Gabapentin is some of the time endorsed to oversee conditions like fretful legs disorder that can disrupt rest. The ideal result is an improvement in rest quality and the decrease of rest aggravations. Assessment includes

surveying changes in rest examples, length, and emotional reports of rest quality.

4. Diminished uneasiness or temperament adjustment. In certain occurrences, gabapentin might be recommended to oversee uneasiness issues or balance out state of mind in specific circumstances. The ideal result is a decrease in uneasiness side effects or mind-set vacillations. Assessment incorporates surveying changes in nervousness levels, mind-set steadiness, and by and large close to home prosperity.

5. Upgraded usefulness. The objective of gabapentin treatment is to work on a patient's general usefulness and personal satisfaction. Assessment includes surveying changes in the patient's capacity to perform everyday exercises, participate in friendly collaborations, and take part in leisure activities or work.

6. Limited secondary effects. Assessing the event and seriousness of secondary effects related with gabapentin is urgent. The ideal result is the counteraction or moderation of aftereffects, like sleepiness, tipsiness, or gastrointestinal side effects. Medical services suppliers evaluate the

presence and effect of aftereffects through quiet reports and objective perceptions.

7. Treatment adherence. Assessment likewise includes surveying the patient's adherence to the endorsed gabapentin routine. The ideal result is steady and legitimate utilization of the drug as trained. Medical services suppliers might ask about medicine adherence, survey reorder history, or utilize different measures to decide consistence.

What is Acetaminophen?

Acetaminophen, otherwise called paracetamol in numerous nations, is a typical over-the-counter pain killer and fever minimizer. It is the dynamic fixing in numerous items like Tylenol. Acetaminophen works by impeding the development of specific synthetic substances in the body that cause agony and irritation. It is for the most part thought to be protected when taken as coordinated, yet taking an excess of can cause liver harm. It is essential to peruse and adhere to the mark guidelines while taking acetaminophen and not surpass the suggested measurement. It ought to likewise be involved with alert in mix with liquor or different drugs.

Nonexclusive Name

acetaminophen

Brand Names

Acetaminophen is the dynamic fixing in numerous over-the-counter (OTC) meds and is accessible under different brand names. The absolute most normal brand names of acetaminophen items include:

- Tylenol
- Abenol
- Acamol
- Acephen
- Acet
- Kids Feverhalt
- Datril
- Fortolin

Newborn child's Feverall

- Liquiprin
- Mapap
- Ofirmev (injectable structure)
- Panadol
- Pediaphen
- Pediatrix
- Taminol

- Tempra

It is essential to take note of that this rundown may not be thorough and there may be other brand names for acetaminophen relying upon the nation or locale.

Drug Order of Acetaminophen

The medication arrangement of acetaminophen is:

Restorative Class

- antipyretics. Acetaminophen is an antipyretic, and that implies it decreases fever.
- nonopioid analgesics. It is likewise a pain relieving, and that implies it assuages torment.

Signs and Remedial Impacts

Acetaminophen is demonstrated for the alleviation of gentle to direct agony and fever. A portion of the normal circumstances for which it is utilized include:

Cerebral pains and headaches. Acetaminophen is by and large viewed as a protected and powerful treatment for gentle to direct cerebral pains, yet it may not be as compelling for serious headaches.

Toothaches. It can likewise be utilized to alleviate torment brought about by toothaches. It works by hindering the development of specific synthetic substances in the body that causes torment and aggravation. It is by and large thought to be a protected and successful treatment for gentle to direct toothaches. Notwithstanding, it is critical to take note of that toothaches can be brought about by different fundamental circumstances and may require dental treatment.

Feminine spasms. Acetaminophen is likewise viewed as a protected and successful treatment for gentle to direct feminine spasms. A few examinations have proposed that taking acetaminophen consistently during the feminine time frame can diminish the seriousness of issues. Notwithstanding, it is vital to take note of that feminine spasms can be brought about by different basic circumstances and may require clinical treatment.

Back torment. During back-torment eruptions, an over-the-counter pain killer, for example, acetaminophen can help through. Medical care suppliers frequently propose first difficult acetaminophen since it is gentler on the stomach, despite the fact that NSAIDs will quite often turn out better for back torment.

Sore throat. Ibuprofen (Advil, Motrin) is a liked over-the-counter (OTC) medication for treating an irritated throat. In any case, it may not be the most secure decision for individuals with specific medical issue, similar to coronary illness and kidney issues. Acetaminophen (Tylenol) might be a more secure throat torment treatment for individuals who can't take ibuprofen.

Cold and influenza side effects. Ibuprofen and acetaminophen can ease cold-related side effects like migraincs, ear infections, and joint agony. For certain individuals, acetaminophen is the most effective way to lessen specific cold and influenza side effects. For other people, ibuprofen gets the job done.

Fevers. Acetaminophen is essentially used to lessen fever and agony. It is an over-the-counter medication, meaning it tends to be purchased without a specialist's solution.

Component of Activity

Acetaminophen is an over-the-counter pain killer and fever minimizer. Its component of activity isn't completely perceived, yet it is remembered to work by hindering the creation of prostaglandins, which are substances in the body that add to agony and irritation. Moreover, it additionally influences the movement of specific synapses in the mind that are engaged with the view of torment. It has no mitigating properties.

Insurances and Contraindications

Acetaminophen is for the most part thought to be protected when taken as coordinated, however there are a few safeguards and contraindications to know about.

A portion of the insurances include:

Overdosage. Go too far can be perilous and possibly lethal, so it is essential to follow the suggested measurements and not surpass the most extreme everyday portion.

Hepatic or Renal illness. People with liver or kidney illness ought to utilize alert while taking acetaminophen, as it is processed by the liver and discharged by the kidneys.

Liquor abuse. Individuals who polish off at least three cocktails day to day ought to try not to take acetaminophen.

Sensitivity. Acetaminophen ought to be involved with alert in individuals with a background marked by sensitivities, asthma, or other breathing issues.

Acetaminophen is contraindicated in specific circumstances, for example,

Touchiness. It ought not be utilized in individuals who are hypersensitive to acetaminophen or any of its latent fixings.

Certain mixtures. Items containing liquor, aspartame, saccharin, sugar, or tartrazine ought to be kept away from in patients who have touchiness or narrow mindedness to these mixtures.

Hepatic or Renal sickness. It ought to be stayed away from in individuals with extreme liver sickness; lower ongoing dosages are suggested.

Different drugs. It ought not be utilized in mix with different meds that contain acetaminophen, as it can build the gamble of excess.

Warfarin. It ought not be taken by individuals who are taking blood-diminishing meds like warfarin, as it might expand the gamble of dying.

Liquor addiction. Constant liquor misuse or blending a lot of liquor with any acetaminophen (or a lot of acetaminophen with any liquor) can make the evacuation of this substance considerably more troublesome. The overabundance substance goes after the liver. This can cause extreme liver harm.

Unhealthiness. Malnourished people are at expanded hazard of acetaminophen hepatotoxicity.

Pregnancy. Use in pregnancy provided that obviously required.

Lactation. Acetaminophen is a decent decision for absence of pain, and fever decrease in nursing moms. Sums in milk are considerably less than portions generally given to babies. Use carefully for IV.

Drug Communications

While directing acetaminophen, the medical caretaker ought to think about the accompanying medication communications:

Drug-Medication

Acetaminophen (Tylenol) can cooperate with a few different meds, including blood thinners, certain antidepressants, and certain anti-microbials. It can likewise communicate with liquor, prompting an expanded gamble of liver harm.

Constant high-portion acetaminophen (>2 g/day) may expand the gamble of draining with warfarin (INR shouldn't surpass 4).

Hepatotoxicity is added substance with other hepatotoxic substances, including liquor.

Simultaneous utilization of isoniazid, rifampin, rifabutin, phenytoin, barbiturates, and carbamazepine may build the gamble of acetaminophen-actuated liver harm (limit self-drug); these specialists will likewise diminish the remedial impacts of acetaminophen.

Simultaneous utilization of NSAIDs might expand the gamble of antagonistic renal impacts (stay away from ongoing simultaneous use).

Propranolol diminishes digestion and may expand its belongings.

May diminish the impacts of lamotrigine and zidovudine.

Drug-Food

Food varieties high in gelatin, including jams, carbs, and different kinds of cruciferous vegetables, for example, broccoli, Brussels fledglings, cabbage, and others, can repress acetaminophen retention. It is hazy the amount of impact this connection possesses on acetaminophen action.

Liquor might build the gamble of hepatotoxicity.

Acetaminophen can be taken regardless of food. The retention is unaffected by food.

Unfavorable Impacts

Acetaminophen (Tylenol) is by and large thought to be protected when taken as coordinated, yet like all prescriptions, it can cause aftereffects in certain individuals.

A few normal symptoms of acetaminophen include:

CNS: tumult, tension, migraine, weakness, sleep deprivation

Resp: atelectasis, dyspnea

CV: hypertension, hypotension

GI: hepatotoxicity, obstruction, expanded liver catalysts, queasiness, retching

F and E: hypokalemia

GU: renal disappointment

Hemat: neutropenia, pancytopenia

MS: muscle fits, lockjaw

Derm: intense summed up exanthematous pustulosis, steven-johnson disorder, harmful epidermal necrolysis

More uncommon aftereffects include:

- Rash
- Urticaria
- Tingling
- Hives
- Enlarging of the face, lips, tongue, or throat
- Trouble relaxing
- Surprising draining or swelling

In uncommon cases, acetaminophen can cause serious aftereffects, for example, yellowing of the skin or eyes, dim pee, and extreme stomach torment.

Organization Contemplations

Accessible Structures

Acetaminophen is accessible in the accompanying structures:

Enjoyable tablets (natural product, bubblegum, or grape flavor): 80 mg, 160 mg.

Tablets: 160 mg, 325 mg.

Caplets: 325 mg.

Arrangement (berry, natural product, and grape flavor): 100 mg/mL.

Fluid (mint): 160 mg/5 mL.

Solution (grape and cherry flavor): 160 mg/5 mL.

Drops: 160 mg/5 mL.

Suspension: 100 mg/mL, 160 mg/5 mL.

Syrup: 160 mg/5 mL.

Suppositories: 80 mg, 120 mg, 325 mg.

Answer for intravenous imbuement: 1000 mg/100 mL in 100-mL vials.

In blend with: numerous different drugs.

Measurement for Children

PO (Children): 10 - 15 mg/kg/portion each 6 - 8 hr on a case by case basis.

IV (Children Birth - 28 days): 12.5 mg/kg each 6 hr (not to surpass 50 mg/kg [by all routes]).

Rect (Youngsters): 10 - 15 mg/kg/portion each 6 - 8 hr on a case by case basis.

Measurement for Babies

PO (Babies): 10 - 15 mg/kg/portion each 6 hr on a case by case basis (not to surpass 5 dosages/24 hr).

IV (Babies 29 days-2 yr): 15 mg/kg each 6 hr (not to surpass 60 mg/kg/day [by all routes]).

Rect (Newborn children): 10 - 20 mg/kg/portion each 4 - 6 hr on a case by case basis.

Measurements for Kids

Youngsters ≤12 yr shouldn't get >5 PO or rectal dosages/24 hr without informing doctor or other medical services proficient. No portion change required while changing over among IV and PO acetaminophen in kids ≥50 kg.

PO (Kids >12 yr): 325 - 650 mg each 6 hr or 1 g 3-4 times day to day or 1300 mg each 8 hr (not to surpass

Dose for Grown-ups

No portion change is required while changing over among IV and PO acetaminophen in grown-ups.

PO (Grown-ups): 325 - 650 mg each 6 hr or 1 g 3-4 times day to day or 1300 mg each 8 hr (not to surpass 3 g or 2 g/24 hr in patients with hepatic/renal debilitation).

IV (Grown-ups ≥50 kg): 1000 mg each 6 hr or 650 mg each 4hr (not to surpass 1000 mg/portion, 4 g/day [by all routes], and under 4 hr dosing stretch).

IV (Grown-ups <50 kg): 15 mg/kg each 6 hr or 12.5 mg/kg each 4 hr (not to surpass 15 mg/kg/portion [up to 750 mg/dose], 75 mg/kg/day [up to 3750 mg/day] [by all routes], and under 4 hr dosing span).

Rect (Grown-ups): 325 - 650 mg each 4-6 hr on a case by case basis or 1 g 3-4 times/day (not to surpass 4 g/24 hr).

Pharmacokinetics

Assimilation. Acetaminophen is quickly ingested from the gastrointestinal lot, with top plasma fixations happening inside 30-an hour of oral organization. Rectal assimilation is variable. Intravenous organization brings about complete bioavailability.

Circulation. Broadly conveyed. Crosses the placenta; enters bosom milk in low focuses.

Digestion and Discharge. 85 - 95% utilized by the liver (CYP2E1 catalyst framework). The medication is used basically in the liver by formation with glucuronide and sulfate, and less significantly by oxidation to N-acetyl-p-benzoquinone imine (NAPQI), which can cause harmfulness in high dosages. Most of the utilized medication is discharged in the pee, with just a little piece discharged in the defecation. Metabolites might be poisonous in glut circumstances.

Half-life. Youngsters: 7 hr; Babies and Kids: 3 - 4 hr; Grown-ups: 1 - 3 hr. As a rule, the half-existence of acetaminophen is 1 - 4 hours. This implies that it requires 1 - 4 hours for half of the medication to be wiped out from the body. The disposal half-existence of acetaminophen is more limited in sound grown-ups, with a middle of 2 hours and a scope of 1 - 4 hours, and somewhat longer in youngsters, the old, and people with liver or kidney brokenness.

Nursing Contemplations for Acetaminophen

It is vital to take note of that acetaminophen ought not be utilized as a substitute for clinical treatment, and it ought to be involved with alert in patients with liver or kidney illness. It ought to likewise be involved with alert in mix with different drugs, particularly those that may likewise influence the liver. While controlling acetaminophen to patients, a few nursing contemplations ought to be considered.

Nursing Evaluation

There are a few significant parts of a nursing evaluation for a patient taking acetaminophen, including:

1. Evaluate the patient's aggravation level prior to controlling the prescription.

Surveying a patient's degree of torment prior to directing acetaminophen is a significant nursing thought. This will assist the medical care supplier with deciding the fitting measurement of the drug.

2. Survey generally speaking wellbeing status and liquor use prior to overseeing acetaminophen.

Patients who are malnourished or constantly misuse liquor are at higher gamble of creating hepatotoxicity with ongoing utilization of common portions of this medication.

3. Evaluate the patient's aggravation level utilizing fitting instruments.

Different instruments can be utilized to evaluate a patient's aggravation level, like the Visual Simple Scale (VAS), the Numeric Rating Scale (NRS), and the Wong-Pastry specialist FACES Agony Rating Scale. These instruments permit the patient to rate their aggravation on a scale, generally from 0-10, with 0 showing no aggravation and 10 demonstrating the most exceedingly terrible aggravation possible.

4. Evaluate the sum, recurrence, and sort of medications taken in patients self-curing, particularly with OTC medications.

Delayed utilization of acetaminophen expands the gamble of unfriendly hepatic and renal impacts. For momentary use, joined portions of acetaminophen and salicylates shouldn't surpass the suggested portion of either drug given alone. Try not to surpass most extreme everyday portion of acetaminophen while thinking about all courses of organization and all mix items containing acetaminophen.

5. Screen the patient's reaction to the prescription.

It is likewise essential to take note of that aggravation evaluation ought to be performed consistently and to screen the patient's reaction to the drug over the span of treatment to guarantee that the medicine is actually dealing with the patient's aggravation and to make any fundamental acclimations to the dose or treatment plan.

6. Evaluate the patient's sensitivities and past responses to prescriptions prior to regulating acetaminophen.

The patient's sensitivities and past responses to meds are significant interesting points to keep away from expected unfavorably susceptible responses. Acetaminophen might cause Stevens-Johnson condition. Suspend treatment if rash (blushing of skin, rankles, and separation of upper surface of skin stripping) or on the other hand whenever joined by fever, general disquietude, exhaustion, muscle or joint throbs, rankles, oral sores, conjunctivitis, hepatitis, or potentially eosinophilia.

7. Screen patients with liver or kidney brokenness for possible unfriendly impacts and change the dose likewise.

People with liver or kidney illness ought to be extra cautious while taking acetaminophen, as it is processed by the liver and discharged by the kidneys.

8. Evaluate fever; note the presence of related signs (diaphoresis, tachycardia, and discomfort).

Evaluating a patient's fever is a significant nursing thought while controlling acetaminophen. Fever is a typical side effect of numerous sicknesses and can be a mark of a basic contamination or condition.

Nursing Determination

A few nursing judgments might be fitting for a patient taking acetaminophen, contingent upon the patient's singular circumstance. A few models include:

Intense agony connected with irritation, injury, or medical procedure, as proven by verbalization of torment and physiologic pointers, for example, expanded pulse and circulatory strain.

Hyperthermia connected with aggravation, as confirmed by an expansion in internal heat level higher than the ordinary reach.

Inadequate information in regards to the protected utilization of acetaminophen, as proven by the patient's absence of comprehension of the suggested measurement, possible secondary effects, and connections with different prescriptions.

Ineffectual wellbeing upkeep connected with insufficient agony the board, as confirmed by the patient's verbalization of continuous torment and unfortunate rest quality.

Assuming the patient is associated with acetaminophen glut, the accompanying nursing analysis might be proper:

Risk for injury connected with extreme utilization of acetaminophen, as confirmed by the patient's set of experiences of surpassing the suggested dose or utilization of numerous items containing acetaminophen.

Risk for hindered liver capability connected with unnecessary utilization of acetaminophen, as proven by the patient's set of experiences of surpassing the suggested dose or utilization of different items containing acetaminophen.

It's critical to take note of that nursing analyze depend on the patient's particular circumstance, and a far reaching evaluation ought to be finished to recognize the right determination.

Acetaminophen Nursing Mediations

While really focusing on a patient taking acetaminophen, there are a few nursing intercessions that can be carried out to guarantee the protected and viable utilization of the prescription:

1. Regulate the medicine in the proper measurements, as recommended by a medical care supplier.

Acetaminophen is by and large viewed as protected when taken as coordinated, yet t is critical to follow the suggested measurements and not surpass the most extreme everyday portion to stay away from excess and expected liver harm. Go too far can be risky and possibly lethal.

2. Try not to mistake Tylenol for Tylenol PM.

Tylenol PM is a mix medication used to treat intermittent sleep deprivation related with minor a throbbing painfulness. Tylenol PM isn't so much for use in that frame of mind without agony, or rest issues that happen frequently.

3. Try not to surpass the greatest suggested everyday portion of acetaminophen when joined with narcotics

While managing acetaminophen in mix with narcotics, it is vital to know about the greatest suggested everyday portion of acetaminophen. Surpassing the greatest suggested everyday portion can build the gamble of liver harm. The most extreme suggested everyday portion of acetaminophen is 4,000 milligrams each day for grown-ups and 90 milligrams for every kilogram each day for youngsters. It is vital to take note of that this is the greatest suggested portion when taken alone and when joined with narcotics, the most extreme suggested day to day portion of acetaminophen might be lower.

4. Manage acetaminophen with a full glass of water.

Acetaminophen can be taken while starving, however make a point to encourage the patient to take it with a full glass of water to stay away from a steamed stomach.

5. Acetaminophen might be taken with food or while starving.

Acetaminophen can be taken with food or while starving however consistently with a full glass of water. Now and again, taking the prescription with food can diminish any steamed stomach that might happen.

6. Intravenous Organization

Discontinuous Implantation

For 1000 mg portion. Embed vented IV set through the septum of a 100 mL vial; might be controlled minus any additional weakening.

For portions <1000 mg. Pull out the suitable portion from the vial and spot it in a different unfilled, sterile holder for IV mixtures. Place little volume pediatric portions up to 60 mL in a needle and regulate through needle siphon. The arrangement is clear and dreary; don't direct stained arrangements or contain particulate matter. Direct inside 6 hrs of breaking the vial seal.

Rate. Mix more than 15 min. Screen the finish of mixture to forestall air embolism, particularly assuming that acetaminophen is the essential imbuement.

Y-Site Similarity

buprenorphine, butorphanol, cefoxitin, ceftriaxone, clindamycin, D5W, dexamethasone, dexmedetomidine, D10W, D5/LR, D5/0.9% NaCl, diphenhydramine, dolasetron, droperidol, esmolol, fentanyl, gentamicin, granisetron, heparin, hydrocortisone, hydromorphone, ketorolac, LR, lidocaine, lorazepam, mannitol, meperidine, methylprednisolone, metoclopramide, midazolam, morphine, nalbuphine, 0.9% NaCl, ondansetron, oxytocin, piperacillin/tazobactam, potassium chloride, prochlorperazine, ranitidine, sufentanil, vancomycin.

Y-Site Contrariness

acyclovir, chlorproma-zine, diazepam, metronidazole.

Added substance Contrariness

Try not to blend in with different prescriptions.

Patient Training and Instructing

1. Instruct patients on the protected utilization of acetaminophen, including the significance of not surpassing the suggested measurements.

Go too far can be risky and possibly lethal, so it is vital to follow the suggested measurement and not surpass the most extreme everyday portion. Ongoing unreasonable utilization of

4 g/day (2 g in persistent heavy drinkers) may prompt hepatotoxicity, renal, or heart harm.

2. Encourage patients to look for clinical consideration in the event that they experience indications of excess, like queasiness, heaving, loss of hunger, perspiring, disarray, or yellowing of the skin or eyes.

Go too far can be perilous and possibly deadly.

3. Guidance the patient to not take acetaminophen longer than ten days and youngsters not longer than five days except if coordinated by a medical care proficient.

Taking an excess of acetaminophen can hurt the liver, once in a while prompting a liver transfer or passing. The body separates a large portion of the acetaminophen in an ordinary portion and dispenses with it in the pee. Yet, a portion of the medication is changed over into a side-effect that is poisonous to the liver.

4. Encourage patients to take the prescription with food or a glass of water.

Acetaminophen can be taken while starving, yet try to encourage the patient to take it with a full glass of water to limit stomach upset.

5. Encourage the patient to suspend acetaminophen and inform the medical care proficient assuming rash happens.

Acetaminophen may only from time to time cause serious skin responses. Side effects might incorporate skin blushing, rash, rankles, and the upper surface of the skin might become isolated from the lower layers.

6. Educate patients to check the name regarding different meds they are taking, as acetaminophen is in many cases tracked down in mix with different medications.

Acetaminophen (Tylenol) can cooperate with a few different prescriptions, including blood thinners, certain antidepressants, and certain anti-toxins. It can likewise cooperate with liquor, prompting an expanded gamble of liver harm.

7. Encourage the patient to keep away from liquor while taking the medicine.

Blending liquor in with any acetaminophen can make the evacuation of this substance significantly more troublesome. The overabundance substance goes after the liver. This can cause extreme liver harm.

8. Examine with the patient the likely dangers of unnecessary utilization of acetaminophen over a significant stretch of time.

Teaching patients about the possible dangers of inordinate utilization of acetaminophen over a significant stretch of time is a significant nursing thought. Acetaminophen is used principally in the liver and in high dosages, it can cause harmfulness, prompting liver harm.

9. Illuminate the patients with diabetes that acetaminophen might modify the aftereffects of blood glucose observing. Encourage patient to advise medical services proficient in the event that changes are noted.

Acetaminophen obstructs persistent glucose screen (CGM) detecting, bringing about dishonestly raised CGM glucose values in the two sensors as of now supported by the U.S. Food and Medication Organization (FDA).

10. Encourage the patient to counsel medical care proficient in the event that distress or fever isn't let

by routine dosages free from this medication or on the other hand assuming fever is more noteworthy than 39.5°C (103°F) or endures longer than three days.

Infections are incredibly heat safe which is the reason viral contaminations ordinarily bring about extremely high temperatures and are not handily controlled with ordinary fever drug like acetaminophen. For instance, dengue fever side effects don't decrease completely with acetaminophen or paracetamol.

11. For Youngsters

Encourage the guardians or parental figures to actually take a look at centralizations of fluid arrangements.

All OTC single-fixing acetaminophen fluid items currently arrive in a solitary grouping of 160 mg/5 mL. Blunders have brought about serious liver harm.

Have guardians or parental figures decide the right definition and portion for their youngster in light of the kid's age or weight, and exhibit how to gauge it utilizing a proper estimating gadget.

Assessment and Wanted Results

The ideal result of utilizing acetaminophen is relief from discomfort and fever decrease. The medication's viability can be assessed by estimating the patient's decrease in torment and fever subsequent to taking the medicine. Moreover, the security of the medication can be assessed by checking for any secondary effects or unfriendly responses that might happen. Standard checking of liver capability tests is expected for long haul use. A medical care proficient ought to be counseled for proper use and dosing.

Made in the USA
Middletown, DE
12 October 2023

40609137R10106